THE PURSUIT OF LIFE

The Pursuit of Life

The Promise and Challenge of Palliative Care

EDITED BY ROBERT FINE AND JACK LEVISON
WITH KELSEY SPINNATO

Foreword by Diane Meier

The Pennsylvania State University Press
University Park, Pennsylvania

Library of Congress Cataloging-in-Publication Data

Names: Fine, Robert (Robert Lee), editor. | Levison, John R., editor.
Title: The pursuit of life : the promise and challenge of palliative care / edited
  by Robert Fine and Jack Levison ; with Kelsey Spinnato.
Description: University Park, Pennsylvania : The Pennsylvania State University
  Press, [2023] | Includes bibliographical references and index.
Summary: "Examines crucial concerns in palliative care, including the proper
  balance between comfort and cure for the patient, the integration of
  spiritual well-being, and the challenges of providing care in the absence of
  basic medical services and supplies"—Provided by publisher.
Identifiers: LCCN 2022042553 | ISBN 9780271094403 (hardback) | ISBN
  9780271094410 (paperback)
Subjects: LCSH: Palliative treatment.
Classification: LCC R726.8 .P87 2023 | DDC 616.02/9—dc23/eng/20220913
LC record available at https://lccn.loc.gov/2022042553

Published by The Pennsylvania State University Press,
University Park, PA 16802–1003

The Pennsylvania State University Press is a member of the Association of
University Presses.

It is the policy of The Pennsylvania State University Press to use acid-free paper.
Publications on uncoated stock satisfy the minimum requirements of American
National Standard for Information Sciences—Permanence of Paper for Printed
Library Material, ANSI Z39.48–1992.

To Richard "Richie" Payne, MD
August 24, 1951–January 3, 2019

Dr. Richard Payne was among the foremost leaders and scholars in the field of palliative care, having served as director of palliative medicine both at MD Anderson and Memorial Sloan Kettering before directing the Duke Institute on Care at the End of Life. Like so many who wrote for this volume, Richard was a scholar par excellence and was already working with Jack and Bob on a medicine in humanities project when Jack conceived of this book. Bob had worked with Richard for a couple of decades, Jack only for a few years—and we both agreed he would be a wonderful contributor to this book. Richard graciously agreed, and we discussed an essay dealing with racial disparities in end-of-life care, a physician's perspective on the role of spirituality in palliative medicine, or frankly any other palliative care topic he wished to write about! We knew that whatever he might submit, it would be a superb contribution to the collection. Upon learning of his unexpected death, we, along with several of our colleagues, immediately realized that the work should be dedicated to him—to his wisdom, wit, and calming, even angelic, smile. We take solace in knowing the world is a better place and the field of palliative medicine a better discipline because of his presence.

CONTENTS

FOREWORD

Most books about palliative care document the major illnesses afflicting humans, the sources of suffering and distress that these illnesses may cause, and how best to identify and remediate such suffering. This content is essential and necessary, but it misses profound truths about palliative care. Truths that commonly result in the curiosity and wrinkled brows of people I meet when I tell them what I actually do. Truths that go well beyond a list of symptoms and their treatments, beyond scripts for assessing patient wishes, and beyond the growing and varied structures that contain and enable this approach to care in hospitals, nursing homes, and community settings.

These truths—perhaps they are not entirely self-evident—have to do with what palliative care teams actually do and experience in a day's work. The conscious confrontation with finitude. A willingness to recognize and remain present with suffering. A determination to lessen pain and suffering. An honest acknowledgment of the limitations of human agency and control, both within medicine and all of life. And the recognition that love and connection—the *I and Thou*[1] of the relationship between clinician and patient—contains the essence of healing. These relationships are, after all, what give clinical practice, and life itself, rich and enduring meaning.[2]

This book digs into the reality—the lived human experience—behind the evidence and the science and the knowledge of palliative care. Reading these essays broadened my conception of my profession, connecting it to the work of poets, readers and teachers, philosophers and ethicists, and pastors. I am not a religious person in the traditional sense, but this book filled me with a sense of the transcendence of our daily experience in palliative care. When people ask me what I do, now I will refer them to this book, as rich and challenging and complex as the work itself.

DIANE E. MEIER

AUGUST 25, 2021

NOTES

1. Buber 1937.

2. Berger 1967.

WORKS CITED

Berger, J. 1967. *A Fortunate Man*. New York: Holt, Rinehart and Winston.

Buber, M. 1937. *I and Thou*. Translated by R. G. Smith. Edinburgh: T&T Clark.

ACKNOWLEDGMENTS

This unique volume epitomizes the power of cooperation. Funding for it came from no fewer than four sources: the Shohet Scholars Program of the International Catacomb Society; a Scholarly Outreach Award from Perkins School of Theology, Southern Methodist University; the W. J. A. Power Chair of Old Testament Interpretation and Biblical Hebrew at Perkins School of Theology; and the Baylor Scott and White Foundation. To each of these we are indebted; for each of these we are grateful.

The occasion for this volume came initially from Dr. Mauro Ferrari, who spearheaded the Palliative Care and Spirituality for Life Conference on September 16–18, 2018. That conference is another exemplar of cooperation. The Roman Catholic Church's Pontifical Academy for Life, the University of Texas MD Anderson Cancer Center, and Houston Methodist Hospital together contributed to this remarkable conference, which coincided as well with the Marialuisa Lectureship for Life, a history of which can be found in the appendix to this book.

We are indebted as well to the good people at Penn State University Press, who championed this project, though it does not quite fit into the usual parameters of most books. Patrick Alexander, Kendra Boileau, Josie DiNovo, Cate Fricke, Brian Beer, and John Morris deserve our thanks for transforming our proposal into an actual book.

Finally, Kelsey Spinnato, a doctoral candidate at Southern Methodist University, lent her considerable experience of three years in the publishing world to this volume. We can say with a degree of certainty—and without hyperbole—that this book might not have seen the light of day without her expertise and efficiency. Unflappable and affable, Kelsey wrestled this book into its current form, and to her we both express our untrammeled gratitude.

Introduction

Robert Fine and Jack Levison

A THIRD-GRADE EPIPHANY

I (Bob) recall my daughter's third-grade Bring-Your-Father-to-School day. One after another, students grasped their fathers' hands, shuffled to the front of the classroom, and explained what this or that father did for a living. "This is my dad. He's a doctor. He fixes broken bones," said one little boy, holding the hand of an orthopedist. "This is my father. He builds houses," said another, grasping the thick hand of his father. "This is my father. He's a surgeon. He fixes people's hearts," said one daughter while holding a thoracic surgeon's hand, which, on any other day, would deftly maneuver tools to replace a broken valve or bypass a clogged artery.

My daughter nervously grabbed my hand as we strolled to the front of the class. "This is my daddy. He helps people die." The children stared dumbfounded. My medical colleagues, the orthopedist and thoracic surgeon, let out unguarded chuckles. "Sweetheart," I said, "I think your class might understand better if we say I treat pain in patients who are really, really, really sick." I looked to the teacher for guidance and, seeing none, told the class, "And sometimes, kids, the patients I treat are so sick that they die. I am very sad when that happens."

Palliative care specialists do not set broken bones or bypass clogged arteries. Rather, they lessen all sorts of pain, including the total pain, the *total suffering*, of those facing the most serious of illnesses. They do not, like so many medical specialists, organize their labor around various organs of the body. Neurology for the brain. Hepatology for the liver. Nephrology for the kidneys. Cardiology for the heart. Ophthalmology for the eyes. Orthopedics for the bones. Pediatrics for the young. Geriatrics for the old. But palliative care? What does the palliativist do, if not to rescue, not to cure?

A FLEDGLING DISCIPLINE

In 1543, Bartholemew Traheron, who would hold posts as member of Parliament, dean of Chichester Cathedral, and canon at Windsor Castle, translated into English *Practica in arte chirurgica copiosa*, a massive nine-volume surgical compendium by Giovanni da Vigo, the official surgeon of Pope Julius II. In a single line, Traheron, translating Vigo's observations on the treatment of a canker—what we would today call an ulcerated mass—captured a distinction that has propelled and plagued the art and science of medicine for centuries: "We wyll speake of his cure aswel eradicatyue as palliatyue." Too often in modern times, we are asked if the goal of medicine is eradication or palliation. Cure or comfort. Might this be a false dichotomy? Might not the goal of medicine, as Giovanni da Vigo, half a millennium ago, suggested, be both curative and palliative?

Though the distinction is old, the discipline of palliative care is new. Specialty certification in hospice and palliative medicine was not offered by the American Board of Medical Specialties and the Accreditation Council for Graduate Medical Education until 2006—though the gestation period began more than half a century earlier. Many pioneers, some of whom are authors in this book, nurtured this new discipline, starting with Dame Cicely Saunders, the English social worker, nurse, and physician who spearheaded the modern hospice movement, and Balfour Mount, the Canadian urologic cancer surgeon most often credited with founding the palliative care movement.[1]

Unfortunately and too often, the terms "palliative care" and "hospice" are confused with each other, leading at times to patient harm, especially when physicians and patients delay referral to palliative care because they believe it is identical with hospice. To avoid this confusion, it is best to think first of supportive palliative care, which ideally serves the sickest 5 to 10 percent of the population in any given year. This sort of care, measured in a span of months to years, should be offered *early*, alongside efforts to slow down, cause remission of, or even eradicate and thus cure the primary disease.

Supportive palliative care can benefit patients by relieving complex suffering—not only physical symptoms like pain or nausea, but emotional symptoms like depression or anxiety, the social suffering of the patient's family, and even spiritual distress. But, as a growing body of literature suggests, early supportive palliative care can also improve survival, at least among metastatic cancer patients.[2] The benefits of *early* palliative care are so compelling that the American Society of Clinical Oncology recommends such services within eight weeks of the diagnosis of metastatic, stage IV, cancer.[3]

The second and more familiar type of palliative care is known as hospice care. Hospice, which first arrived in the United States in 1975, serves especially the dying, who make up less than 1 percent of the population in any given year. Sometimes hospice begins only hours or days prior to death, but typically it spans a time frame of weeks to a few months. With a few exceptions, hospice, unlike supportive palliative care, does not begin until a patient and physician conclude that further attempts to slow the progression of disease are neither possible nor desirable.

The palliativist's job, whether working in supportive palliative care or in hospice, is not principally to diagnose and treat *disease*, but rather to diagnose and treat the *suffering*, the dis-ease, that inevitably falls on the shoulders of those who face serious illness. The meaning of the noun "diagnosis" is related to the Greek verb *diagnōskein*, to decide, to determine, to distinguish. Diagnosis of disease relies on the hard sciences and is an essential, indispensable tool, but not the sole or even sufficient tool for the care of the whole person. A second sort of diagnosis, the diagnosis of human suffering, is also necessary. Paul Kalanithi, a neurosurgeon who died of cancer at the age of thirty-seven, embraces this distinction in his memoir, *When Breath Becomes Air*: "Science may provide the most useful way to organize empirical, reproducible data, but its power to do so is predicated on its inability to grasp the most central aspects of human life: hope, fear, love, hate, beauty, envy, honor, weakness, striving, suffering, virtue."[4] If the diagnosis of disease is an effort to ensure *that* we live, the diagnosis of suffering through palliative care is an effort to enrich *how* we live, especially in the shadow of death.

No single definition of palliative care, therefore, will do. No sterile job description will suffice. Because not all disease can be cured, nor all pain eradicated with a laser, scalpel, radiation beam, chemical, genetic, or other biological manipulation, palliative care experts coordinate, collaborate, and cooperate in multidisciplinary teams to palliate, to cloak, to relieve total pain. Palliative care is, in essence, the diagnosis and management of suffering, the *total* suffering of physical, social, emotional, and spiritual pain. Palliativists care for the most seriously ill among us. Story after story in this volume attests to the complex, multidisciplinary, global, and occasionally heroic effort to manage that total suffering.

AN ANCIENT STORY OF PAIN

A preoccupation with pain is nothing new. It goes back to the beginning—as far back as Genesis, in the Bible's opening story. The intimacy of a potter-God's lips pressed against a freshly formed human figure, poised to blow breath within, brings the promise of unending love. This is wildly exciting if somewhat awkward. Yet even before that first kiss of life, we are alerted to the underside of creation: Adam—human—is dust from the ground. The new life, full and rich and pulsing with potential, is blown into someone who, in short measure, will be condemned to return to the earth, ashes to ashes, dust to dust.

But not before he—and she—knows the story of pain. They will know physical pain, these first two, but not in an antiseptic sort of way, not neatly diagnosed and dispensed with. The curses of everyman and everywoman— they are not yet named as individuals, so their story is *our* story—are expressed by the resonant Hebrew word *itsavon* (ʿiṣṣābôn). The man and woman, both, will know *itsavon*. The woman will experience *itsavon* when she is in labor. The man, too, will experience *itsavon* when he labors in the field. Man and woman both labor, both know *itsavon*, he to wrest fruit from the soil and she to wrest fruit from the womb—both, in antiquity, doubtful and difficult ventures.[5]

In the Bible's opening scene, then, there is no divvying up of pain. The broad-shouldered first word for the *man's* pain fuses sweat and toil and grief and loss and hurt with, in the vagaries of antiquity, occasional healthy harvest; the same word for the *woman's* pain fuses sweat and toil and grief and loss and hurt with, in the vagaries of antiquity, occasional joy and life and healthy birth. The scholars who transposed the Hebrew into Greek in ancient Alexandria seem to have understood the density of this first word for pain. They translated the Hebrew words for pain in this story with the Greek words *lupē*, grief, and *stenagmos*, groan. The man would know pain, but not only in his weary back and blistered palms. The woman's pain would transcend the breaching of a cervix. Life, the very first story tells us, is destined to be rife with grief, raw with groans.

Such is a sliver of ancient literature, offering not a clinical diagnosis, as important as that is, but a story to be told, heard, and told back again. A story of pain, of grief, of groaning. A mirror, even, of our own pain a trillion heartbeats later. Siddhartha Mukherjee, in his memoir *The Emperor of All Maladies: A Biography of Cancer*, tells us that "medicine . . . begins with storytelling. . . . Patients tell stories to describe illness; doctors tell stories to understand it. Science tells its own story to explain diseases."[6] The Bible—some of humankind's most ancient literature—begins by telling the story of pain. Relentless and inexorable and all-encompassing. *Total* pain. The first story—and it's meant to be told and heard this way—of *our* pain.

A STORY YET UNFOLDING

I (Jack) moved to Southern Methodist University in 2015 to teach Hebrew Bible, what Christians call the Old Testament. I arrived with modest financial support from the International Catacomb Society perhaps to do something a little different from my prior work. With a history of searing headaches, I resolved to expand our understanding of pain by connecting ancient texts on pain and suffering with modern medical practitioners, whose responsibility it is to palliate pain, especially near the end of life. I was introduced to the palliative care and clinical ethics specialist Bob Fine, who just happened to live down the street from my office. Over several hours of exhilarating front porch conversations, it became obvious, at least to the two of us, that the biblical antiquities professor and the palliativist and ethicist had much to learn from each other about pain and suffering.

Encouraged by the camaraderie I experienced with Bob, I began to gather a small coterie of scholars of antiquity and modern medical practitioners. They were an improbable cluster, by any measure, yet together we met, physicians and scholars, to wrest insight for palliative care from ancient texts on pain. Among them were Joe Calandrino and Joe Fins, both of whom have contributed creative essays to this book; Richard Payne, to whose memory this book is dedicated; and, of course, Bob Fine. We met informally twice in New York City, thanks to the hospitality of Brooke Holmes, Goheen Professor of Classics at Princeton University.

About the same time, a group from Perkins School of Theology at Southern Methodist University visited the Houston Methodist Research Institute. There I met Mauro Ferrari, CEO of the Institute. A few years later, in 2018, Mauro told me that something unprecedented was about to happen. The Roman Catholic Church's Pontifical Academy for Life was planning to hold a conference for the first time on American soil, in collaboration with Houston Methodist Research Institute and the department of palliative, rehabilitation, and integrative medicine at the University of Texas MD Anderson Cancer Center. The foundation of this unprecedented symposium, Palliative Care and Spirituality for Life, would be the Marialuisa Lectureship for Life, the history of which Mauro has chronicled in an appendix to this volume.

I introduced Mauro to Bob Fine, and both of us attended this stunning symposium. I could not help but notice the remarkable lineup of speakers, so I met immediately with Mauro to discuss publication. The speakers, I knew, represented an array of luminaries in the field. So, shortly after the symposium ended, Bob, whom I had asked to coedit the volume, and I gathered contributors, adding one or two who had not attended the symposium, and set about to produce this volume. Like the symposium, this volume is unique, defying any single category and scrambling tidy parameters.

A VOLUME WITH MANY PERSPECTIVES

The first part of this volume, "Palliative Care: Personal Memoirs," consists of personal histories of palliative care from the perspective of some of its pioneers: Constance Dahlin, Eduardo Bruera, Neil MacDonald, and Declan Walsh. Nowhere else is the primal challenge and unfolding promise of palliative care documented so personally and professionally. Nowhere else are so many varied stories of those who forged a new discipline, from the days of Dame Cicely Saunders, recorded. As editors, we have made a good-faith effort to preserve the unique, even idiosyncratic, voices in this section. Dahlin's essay represents a professional history of palliative care from the perspective of nursing. Bruera, MacDonald, and Walsh offer various personal reflections on the emergence of palliative care, with an eye to the institutional and personal challenges early proponents faced. These are unique and influential voices. For these alone, the volume would be worth reading.

The second part of this volume, "Palliative Care: Pain and Suffering," contains essays that might be said to have their home in the burgeoning field of medical humanities. The starting point for Joseph Fins's essay on the nature of time is Tennessee Williams's *The Glass Menagerie*. Kathryn Kirkland offers a slow and thoughtful reading of Jane Kenyon's poem "Coats" in an essay directed to pedagogy. And Joseph Calandrino draws intimate and innovative connections between the ancient playwright Sophocles's *Philoctetes* and the suffering of contemporary patients. Though ranging widely, all three essays in this section are connected by a deft and daring ability to shed light on palliative care through its unlikely association with various bits and pieces of poetry and plays, ancient and modern.

The third part of this volume, "Palliative Care: Essential Issues," is perhaps its most eclectic. Ethicists Robin Lovin and Daniel Sulmasy explore the question of autonomy through two quite different lenses; the locus of Sulmasy's essay is a monastery, while Lovin's focus is various patients, but together they ask the question of what constitutes the good—a thorny inquiry—in the context of pain and suffering. James Cleary and Costantino Benedetti tackle issues related to opioids, though from altogether different perspectives. Benedetti focuses upon an American tragedy, Cleary upon a global crisis. Dominique Monlezun's essay looks to the future, with an eye toward the impact of artificial intelligence on the evolution of palliative care.

The final section, "Palliative Care: The Caregiver," contains various primers for those who accompany men and women who suffer. Andrew Achenbaum, starting with Leo Tolstoy's *The Death of Ivan Ilych*, a book often used to introduce medical students to the phenomena of pain, suffering, and death, offers insights from his own personal journey as a caregiver, providing guidance for others who are or will become caregivers themselves. Courtenay Bruce, Stacy Auld, and Charles Millikan offer an institutional point of view as individuals who have successfully incorporated the spiritual component of care in a nationally renowned hospital. Bettie Hightower offers a grassroots perspective on hospital chaplaincy, while Tullio Proserpio, Elena Pagani Bagliacca, Giovanna Sironi, and Andrea Ferrari tell the story of a remarkable institution in Milan and how chaplains make inroads into the lives of adolescents with cancer. The story of Lucia, who anchors this final essay, is worth telling in any land.

This volume has something to say to a breathtaking array of readers, to any "human merely being" in the face of serious illness, from patients to family members to physicians, and to any other members of the health care team.[7] Pioneers of the field lead us back in an unvarnished way to the matter of origins. Leading researchers, who are shaping approaches to palliative care for the next generation, offer fresh perspectives on topics as diverse as narrative approaches to medicine, the nature of time, and global challenges to palliative care; these essays span the ages, from Sophocles's *Philoctetes* to the promise of artificial intelligence. Ethicists lead us, through anecdotes and analysis, into a discussion of human flourishing and the challenges of individualism in palliative care. Colleagues from Milan introduce us to innovations in an institute devoted exclusively to adolescents with cancer. The breadth of essays is stunning, but the wealth of experience even more so. This volume offers an extraordinary look at palliative care: its history, told through hard-won experience; its challenges, told in institutional, ethical, and global terms; its spiritual dimensions, told from the perspective of spiritual care providers, both professional and volunteer; and its unfolding perspectives, told in ways both practical and innovative.

NOTES

1. The recent publication of Balfour Mount's *Ten Thousand Crossroads: The Path as I Remember It* (2020) deserves mention.

2. Temel et al. 2010; Bakitas et al. 2014; Sullivan et al. 2019.

3. Ferrell et al. 2017.

4. Kalanithi 2016, 170.

5. These words can be found in Genesis 3:16–19.

6. Mukherjee 2010, 390.

7. The language of a "human merely being" is borrowed from E. E. Cummings's "I thank you God for most this amazing."

WORKS CITED

Bakitas, M., T. Tosteson, Z. Li, K. Lyons, J. Hull, Z. Li, J. N. Dionne-Odom, J. Frost, M. Hegel, A. Azuero, T. Ahles, J. R. Rigas, J. M. Pipas, and K. H. Dragnev. 2014. "The ENABLE III Randomized Controlled Trial of Concurrent Palliative Oncology Care." *Journal of Clinical Oncology* 32 (15s): 9512.

Ferrell, B. R., J. S. Temel, S. Temin, E. R. Alesi, T. A. Balboni, E. M. Basch, J. I. Firn, J. A. Paice, J. M. Peppercorn, T. Phillips, E. L. Stovall, C. Zimmermann, and T. J. Smith. 2017. "Integration of Palliative Care into Standard Oncology Care: American Society of Clinical Oncology Clinical Practice Guideline Update." *Journal of Clinical Oncology* 35 (1): 96–112.

Kalanithi, P. 2016. *When Breath Becomes Air.* New York: Random House.

Mount, B. 2020. *Ten Thousand Crossroads: The Path as I Remember It.* Montreal: McGill-Queen's University Press.

Mukherjee, S. 2010. *The Emperor of All Maladies: A Biography of Cancer.* New York: Scribner.

Sullivan, D. R., B. Chan, J. A. Lapidus, L. Ganzini, L. Hansen, P. A. Carney, E. K.

Fromme, M. Marino, S. E. Golden, K. C. Vranas, and C. G. Slatore. 2019. "Association of Early Palliative Care Use with Survival and Place of Death Among Patients with Advanced Lung Cancer Receiving Care in the Veterans Health Administration." *JAMA Oncology* 5 (12): 1702–9.

Temel, J. S., J. A. Greer, A. Muzikansky, E. R. Gallagher, S. Admane, V. A. Jackson, C. M. Dahlin, C. D. Blinderman, J. Jacobsen, W. F. Pirl, J. A. Billings, and T. J. Lynch. 2010. "Early Palliative Care for Patients with Metastatic Non-Small-Cell Lung Cancer." *New England Journal of Medicine* 363:733–42.

Palliative Care

Personal Memoirs

CHAPTER 1

Evolution of Palliative Nursing
Art, Science, and Collaboration

Constance Dahlin

In the corner of a living room, Kate, a woman in her thirties, lies dying of breast cancer. She is weak and mostly bedbound. Her husband, Rick, is struggling to come to terms with her dying and how he will care for their two young children. The home hospice nurse visits frequently to manage pain medications, assist with personal care, and coach Rick. She visits Kate three times a week to assess her physical well-being, including her response to the pain-management plan, and to address how Kate and Rick are doing coping with her illness and the life changes it has and will cause. This includes Kate's changing role as a mother, her wishes for her legacy to her young daughters, and Rick's need for support and help with practical concerns and his fear of being alone. The hospice nurse listens to their hopes and worries, offers suggestions, and encourages the use of the social worker and chaplain. Sometimes the hospice nurse is accompanied by Diana, the chaplain, or Judy, the social worker, allowing the nurse some time alone with Kate as they tend to Rick and vice versa. At the weekly interdisciplinary team meeting, all the team members involved with Kate's care discuss her diagnosis, prognosis, pain and symptom levels, psychological coping, and care needs. Recommendations are made to the oncologist about medications using evidence-based practice. The goal of care is to ensure Kate's comfort to keep her at home, to support Rick to enable him to keep his wife at home, and to offer resources for respite care and support for the children.

Death is our common experience as humans. Throughout human history, a scenario has recurred—a person with a life-ending illness is lying in the middle of the room, surrounded by family. Into current times, there has often been a woman whose role it is to care for or minister to the sick patient (i.e., a nurse). She offers the art of care—individualized physical comfort for pain and symptoms, psychological comfort in providing therapeutic presence to support coping, spiritual care in offering appropriate rituals and therapies in line with faith and culture, and emotional/social care in attending to the patient's changing role in the family, and the changing family itself.

Kate was one of the first patients under my care in 1986. I was a new nurse, having just completed a master of science in nursing in oncology. Cancer was a serious and often life-limiting diagnosis, with few treatments for cure. Many of us felt we needed to have expert knowledge and skills about all aspects of cancer care, to exquisitely manage the many needs of patients from diagnosis to death. There had been a required four-month hospice practicum in the oncology track of my master's program. I felt prepared in my dual roles— being on the front line of delivering novel cancer treatments while serving as midwife and guide to individuals who were dying. When Kate was my patient, care was focused on individuals with cancer, whose options were limited to attempting cure at all costs to the exclusion of comfort or hospice. Today, palliative care serves a broader population of patients who are coping with serious, life-altering illnesses and conditions. Some patients are facing more imminent death, while others cope with life changes associated with serious health impairments. Whatever the circumstances, the basic approach to providing personalized care to enhance quality of life has not changed.

Palliative care is a philosophy that improves the quality of life for patients with serious illness and their families. This goal is achieved through early identification and impeccable assessment of physical, emotional, social, cultural, and spiritual suffering through a team-based creation of a patient-centered treatment plan. This broad multidisciplinary approach includes the patient, the family, and community resources. However, it can be successfully implemented even if family caregivers are unavailable and community resources are limited.[1]

"Palliative care is explicitly recognized as a human right to health," in times of peace or of crisis, and is ideally tailored to the specific needs and preferences of individuals.[2] An interprofessional team ensures that the physical, emotional, social, cultural, and spiritual dimensions of the patient and family are addressed. At its core, the focus of the team is on compassion and respect for human dignity resulting in personal relationships and patient-centered care that also builds on the needs of the family and the resources of their community.

Similar to the other palliative care disciplines, nursing has developed its own art and science of palliative care delivery. Unique to nursing is its prominent role as a frontline care clinician, whether in the home, office, acute care, or long-term care setting. This proximity to the patient necessitates comprehensive assessment of the person and family, responsibility for and advocacy of implementation, evaluation of the treatment plan, and care coordination. The nurse often spends the most time with patients and families and therefore observes family interactions, witnesses a patient's coping, and listens to a patient's most inner thoughts. This promotes a close understanding of the patient and family, establishing the important link of the nurse to the team.

In Kate's situation my ability to assess, evaluate, and implement interventions to manage her care, while bearing witness to the process, gave me the knowledge to advocate for her with the primary team and gave Kate and Rick the confidence I would do so.

HISTORY OF PALLIATIVE NURSING

My choice to start a career in hospice grew out of my work as an oncology nurse. Like all new nurses, I was required to work nights, which I did on a surgical oncology floor. I built my practice on Florence Wald's curriculum, which had been our bible in school. In the still of the night, I had the opportunity to have meaningful conversations with patients and families about their quality of life, their treatment decisions, and their worries and concerns. Often, it was my role to help them find the strength and the words to tell their oncologists that while they appreciated their care, they were ready to stop treatment and focus on family. These exchanges honed my communication skills and my ability to develop authentic nurse-patient relationships. The richness of these conversations solidified my desire at that time to move into the novel arena of hospice. They also became the focus of my advocacy to guide a patient's care according to their wishes.

The art of palliative nursing has a long history. Since Roman times, there have been individuals caring for persons with serious illness.[3] Due to a lack of understanding of disease and illness, many people died at a young age from infection, trauma, or other conditions that are now curable. Notably, death was a ritual accompanied by elaborate traditions.[4] Over time, in Christianity, this resulted in nursing and religion being intertwined as nuns of various denominations ministered to the ill and dying in hostels.[5]

The science of modern palliative nursing begins in the 1800s. Caring for dying individuals was changed by two developments: care for dying soldiers and the founding of hospices to care for terminally ill individuals. Florence Nightingale trained with the Daughters of Charity in Egypt in the 1840s.[6] Along with Mary Seacole, she used that training and observations of how soldiers died in the Crimean War to formulate the foundations of modern nursing principles aimed at the improvement of care. In the United States, Clara Barton continued to use these principles while caring for soldiers in the Civil War.[7] The Irish Sisters of Charity opened several hospices for dying patients: 1879—Lady's Hospice in Dublin; 1900—East End of London; and 1905—St. Joseph's Hospice.[8] In the United States, Sister Rose Lathrop, who had trained as a nurse at the New York Cancer Hospital, opened Hawthorne House for Incurable Cancer as part of her Catholic mission.[9]

In the mid-twentieth century, Cicely Saunders spearheaded the modern hospice movement, the concept of total pain, and exquisite attention to the domains of personhood for individuals who were often ignored because they were at the end of their lives. At St. Luke's Home, Dr. Saunders first began her work in hospice as a nurse, then a social worker.[10] She then became a physician and worked at St. Joseph's Hospice, where she focused on pain management and the concept of total pain. "Looking back, I realize my own Nursing training during World War II showed me the importance of attention to detail and personal commitment. We had nothing but ourselves to give."[11] She then built St. Christopher's Hospice in 1967 and worked to educate nurses. "Nurses were the first to respond to this challenge and remain the core of the personal and professional drive to enable people to find relief, support, and meaning at the end of their lives."[12] However, her principles had yet to be translated into general nursing practice.[13]

In the United States, discussion about death was just beginning with the publication of Dr. Elisabeth Kübler-Ross's *On Death and Dying* in 1969.[14] The foundation of the science of palliative nursing would be accomplished by Dr. Florence Wald, then the dean of Yale School of Nursing.[15] Dr. Wald had studied hospice implementation and understanding the dying process in England. She collaborated with Dr. Kübler-Ross to integrate bereavement principles into end-of-life care. Upon her return, she founded the inpatient Connecticut Hospice in 1974, the first hospice in America.[16]

Dr. Wald then developed an expansive nursing curriculum that emphasized the skills necessary for caring for dying patients, specifically pain and symptom management and communication. She explained, "Hospice care is the epitome of good nursing care. It enables the patient to get through the end of life on their own terms. It is a holistic approach, looking at the patient as an individual, a human being. The spiritual role nurses play in the end of life process is essential to both patients and families."[17] The Hospice Education Program for Nurses was developed at the Yale University School of Nursing in 1981 under the auspices of a health resources grant from the US Department of Health and Human Services.[18] Ten fundamental modules, listed below, were developed by an esteemed interdisciplinary group of nurses, a social worker, a pharmacist, and researchers to develop hospice nursing as a specialty:

- Hospice Care Concepts
- Communication Skills
- Concepts of Death, Dying, and Grief
- Family Dynamics and Family Counseling
- Managing Personal and Organizational Stress in the Care of the Dying
- Understanding the Process of Dying and the Death Event Itself
- Pharmacology
- Pain and Symptom Management
- Interdisciplinary Team Concepts
- Ethical and Legal Issues[19]

The themes of these ten modules have stood the test of time and are as appropriate now as then.

THE MEDICARE HOSPICE BENEFIT AND NURSING

The Medicare Hospice Benefit was formative for nursing. It allowed nurses to utilize all the aspects of nursing practice—communication skills, assessment skills, patient and family education skills, cultural skills, and collaborative skills. There was considerable allure to providing care in the patient's residence, wherever that was, on their own terms. Having considered being a midwife, I was excited that I could be one—albeit to the individuals leaving the world rather than babies entering the world. It was so interesting to watch the concept of hospice develop as an insurance benefit and to work within the regional interpretations of it. To see the possibilities outside the Medicare Benefit, I did a pilgrimage to Connecticut Hospice to experience the concept of hospice in America. As an inpatient facility, it was well resourced and offered the comforts of home and life, as there was even a child-care center on the first floor. Under the auspices of the Hospice Education Institute, I studied hospice in England as it was integrated across health settings, such as out-patient palliative care clinics, presence in adult day care, as well as mobile units. I took a month's sabbatical in Australia to see how care was done in the community and experience a palliative care hospital. I used these concepts when building a program in urban Boston and later in Oregon.

In 1982, the federal government formally recognized the importance of hospice care with passage of the Medicare Hospice Benefit. Under this legislation, terminally ill patients with an expected survival of less than six months could receive hospice care paid for by Medicare. The Medicare Hospice Conditions of Participation (CoPs) clearly delineated the services hospices had to offer patients and families. According to Foster and Corless, Dr. Wald observed, "Hospices grew throughout this nation first as a grassroots healthcare reform effort. . . . Consumers grew to understand that they had the right to influence the quality of their remaining life."[20] It was a health care movement, much like the birth movement, in which individuals took control of a life process, only this time it was the end of life.

Within the Medicare Hospice Benefit and the overall concept of hospice, nursing had a prominent role as a core service. While nurses provide the majority of hospice care within the Medicare Hospice Benefit, they do so with the defined interdisciplinary team. Physicians provide the certification and medical direction of the team and may do occasional home visits. Social workers and chaplains are also important team members. Unfortunately, patients and families often decline the services of the full range of team members, hospice regulations restrict team members to only a few visits, or the number of patients exceeds the bandwidth of the full team to provide service at optimal frequency.

One weakness of the original Medicare Hospice Benefit was that, unlike other countries where hospice and palliative care were a continuum of care, hospice was and is regulated as an insurance benefit rather than a philosophy of care. It requires that patients have a life expectancy of six months or less and they agree to forgo attempts at cure or major life-extending interventions. The limits of hospice were tested in the 1980s with the AIDS epidemic, when a younger population was affected. Both oncology nurses and AIDS nurses proved their expertise in pain and symptom management. However, a significant symptom burden required expensive medications to promote quality of life, not covered by hospice. The result was that many persons with AIDS did not benefit from hospice, and the opportunity to push hospice beyond cancer care was delayed.

FROM HOSPICE TO PALLIATIVE CARE

Like many of my colleagues, I moved from the hospital into the community so I could care for patients at their residence—whether a home, a skilled facility, or an inpatient unit. As expressed by Dr. Florence Wald, I wanted to participate in a consumer movement for dying—similar to the birth movement. As a nurse, I was often the sole professional visiting the patient and family, which necessitated expert knowledge to assess and manage pain and symptoms, along with keen communication skills. I was able to deliver more autonomous and patient-focused care. It was vital to convey information to the team to ensure holistic care and promote collaborative practice. I was quickly challenged by the significant aspects of the AIDS epidemic. I witnessed the many challenges faced by these individuals—the stigma of the disease, the deficiencies of the health system, the ethics of care, and the cost of the new medications. Most distressing, and new to the conversation, was the terrible constellation of the AIDS trajectory, and the desire of these young men who wanted to maintain dignity and exert control in their dying by hastening their death. At the core was quality of life and suffering, and I used all my skills.

In 1986, to promote the specialty of hospice nursing and consistency of practice, the Hospice Nurses Association was established as the first discipline-specific professional hospice and palliative organization in the United States.[21] In 1987, the specialty was formally recognized under the American Nurses Association with the development of the first *Scope and Standards of Hospice Nurse Practice*.[22] This promoted national hospice nursing competencies no matter the size of the hospice program and geographic location of where care was provided. It also promoted better care and established clear expectations for our interdisciplinary colleagues.[23] As a result of this, the National Board for Certification of Hospice Nurses was established in 1993.[24] In 1994, the first specialty palliative care certification examination offered was in hospice nursing,[25] followed by medicine in 1996, social work in 2000, and then by chaplaincy organizations.[26]

MOVEMENT FROM HOSPICE TO PALLIATIVE CARE AND EARLY NURSE PIONEERS

In 1996, Dr. Andrew Billings and I cofounded the Massachusetts General Hospital palliative care service. The first day, all we had was an office with telephones in the middle of the room—no furniture, no coat rack, no chair. We built the service from nothing. We role-modeled collaborative practice and teamwork, bringing many of the principles of hospice care, such as interdisciplinary patient management and team support meetings, to the service. Our purpose was to improve care for seriously ill patients. Our goal was to engage fellow practitioners to recognize the importance of end-of-life care and light their passion. We performed joint patient visits on daily rounds, provided interdisciplinary education sessions, and role-modeled collaborative consultation. Working in a nine-hundred-bed, twenty-six–patient unit hospital, I worked with each of the floors to provide consultation, mentoring, and coaching to the nursing unit leadership and the interdisciplinary team, which included the nurse manager, the clinical nurse specialist, the unit-based nurses, the case managers, the social workers, and the chaplains. Dr. Billings worked with the medical staff and the house staff.

In the early 1970s, a Canadian physician, Dr. Balfour Mount, coined the term "palliative care" to distinguish it from dying houses, bringing hospice concepts into the academic acute care hospital setting in order to improve care of individuals with the most serious illness. This movement was slow to move to the United States. In the 1990s, many professionals (this author included) began to consider the limitations of hospice as it had developed in the United States and who had access to it.[27] What happened to the people with terminal diseases who either did not want hospice nor did not qualify for benefits? How could access to meticulous, interdisciplinary care be ensured for all patients? Some of these feelings were intensified by the movement for medically assisted death (then known as assisted suicide), which made many of us consider if we were doing enough to palliate the suffering of patients with life-limiting illness. This was a seminal moment for American hospice professionals to work together to promote palliative care by using the principles of good care beyond the six months of end-of-life care restrictions offered by hospice. Many hospice professionals moved into larger urban hospitals to promote the art and science of palliative care by establishing programs in academic medical centers.[28] Major funding to develop leaders to improve death and dying in the United States was made possible by George Soros's Open Society Institute—Project on Death in America (PDIA) faculty scholars' program. From 1994 to 2000, there were seventy-eight scholar awards, six of which were nurses.[29]

A monograph from 2000, *Pioneer Programs in Palliative Care: Nine Case Studies*, offers information on some of the initial programs.[30] Interestingly, though these were interdisciplinary teams, including well-known nurse leaders, only two programs list nurses: Jane Morris, nurse coordinator at Mount Sinai Medical Center, and Patrick Coyne, a nurse clinician/administrator at Virginia Commonwealth University. However, nursing had a solid presence at several programs: Nessa Coyle at Memorial Sloan Kettering Cancer Center, Lisa Kramer at Northwestern Memorial Hospital, Pamela Goldstein at Cleveland Clinic, Maureen Lynch at Dana Farber Cancer Institute, and myself at Massachusetts General Hospital. Other nurse leaders in palliative nursing were highlighted in the 2001 monograph *Advanced Practice Nursing: Pioneering Practices in Palliative Care*, including Margaret Campbell at Detroit Receiving Hospital, Patricia Murphy at New Jersey University Hospital, Martha Henderson at University of North Carolina Geriatrics, and Jennifer Gentry at Carver Living Center in North Carolina.[31] We knew each other by name and understood the importance of each of our roles in promoting palliative nursing and creating the future of this specialty practice.

Despite progress in hospice and the establishment of palliative care within the preceding twenty years, other important events painted a complicated picture of dying in America. In 1993, the Decisions Near the End of Life program documented concerns by nurses and physicians about the provision of overly burdensome treatment, overly technological approaches, and inadequate pain management, as well as the fact that nurses felt less empowered to participate in goals of care discussions. This information framed an interdisciplinary approach to professional education to improve care at the end of life.[32] The 1995 SUPPORT study—which had a large, albeit inconsistent, nursing component in its intervention—revealed significant lack of communication and of respect for patient preferences.[33] Specifically, the study highlighted ineffective communication concerning patient wishes at the end of life. Although a nursing intervention was instituted to improve communication, it was inconsistent, and did not have a positive effect. SUPPORT did point out the need for communication skills for physicians and the need for the interdisciplinary team. Second, the 1997 report *Approaching Death: Improving Care at the End of Life*, published by the Institute of Medicine, highlighted poor experiences of dying in America, in spite of stellar technology.[34] Written by an interdisciplinary twelve-member committee—two social workers, six physicians, one nurse, two researchers, and a lawyer—this report recommended specialty palliative care, endorsed appropriate utilization of medications for pain and symptom management, supported financial investment in palliative care, and called for health care provider education, including palliative care principles and practice in both training programs and curriculum textbooks.[35] In the following years, the 2002 Institute of Medicine report *When Children Die* highlighted the need for better care of dying children.[36] The publication of a state-by-state report card on end-of-life care by Last Acts—a newly created entity supported by the Robert Wood Johnson Foundation (RWJF)—painted a dismal depiction of dying in every state and poor palliative care utilization throughout the United States.[37] Clearly, there was work to be done, and nursing would create its own direction.

DEVELOPMENT OF THE SPECIALTY OF HOSPICE AND PALLIATIVE NURSING

As many of us were developing leadership roles within palliative nursing, it was important to role-model specialty practice. The American Nurses Association recognized the specialty practice of palliative nursing in 1987. I took the first specialty nursing examination in hospice and palliative care as a registered nurse in 1994. In 2002, I contributed to writing the scope and standards when the specialty became hospice and palliative nursing. I was also part of a group that developed the clinical competencies that registered nurses (RN) and advanced practice registered nurses (APRN) would be held to. In 2003, having completed a three-year term on the board of the Hospice and Palliative Nurses Association, I felt it was important to lead by example to demonstrate competence and took the first advanced practice specialty examination for hospice and palliative nurses. Although it is not required by the Centers for Medicaid and Medicare Services (CMS) or my state, I have maintained my primary board certification as an adult nurse practitioner and my certification in hospice and palliative nursing as an APRN.

To be successful, it was essential for all disciplines within the field of palliative care to work both together as a team and separately within each discipline to improve education and training of all disciplines in serious illness and end-of-life care, and in so doing, to relieve suffering. With 3.5 million or more nurses representing the largest group of health care professionals, nurses are often on the front line, serving as clinical, educational, and quality-improvement leaders in all serious illness care settings.[38]

In 1997, the Robert Wood Johnson Foundation funded a multifaceted project, Strengthening Nursing Education to Improve End-of-Life Care, which focused on improving nursing knowledge about end of life.[39] The support of RWJF lay in the observation that "training doctors is just part of the story; nurses actually provide most of the professional care for dying people."[40]

Part 1 of the project reviewed nursing textbooks for end-of-life content, which was liberally defined as pain and symptom management or care of the dying patient or spiritual care. With completion of this project in 1999, Dr. Betty Ferrell, Dr. Marcia Grant, and Rose Virani revealed that written content in end-of-life nursing care was nearly nonexistent.[41] The result for nursing education was development of *The Oxford Textbook of Palliative Nursing*. Now in its fifth edition, this nursing text serves as the seminal palliative nursing reference for both RN and APRN practice.

Part 2 of the project examined end-of-life care content in nursing licensing examinations. Research had clearly demonstrated that both RNs and APRNs felt they had inadequate preparation in end-of-life care.[42] This resulted in the creation of baccalaureate education competencies in end-of-life care that were disseminated within the American Association of Colleges of Nursing (AACN) document *Peaceful Death: Recommended Competencies and Curricular Guidelines for End-of-Life Nursing Care*.[43] Palliative and end-of-life content questions appeared within nursing licensure examination. For nearly two decades, these competencies served as the basis for nursing education at both the graduate and the undergraduate level. In 2016, a group of undergraduate faculty, as well as myself, convened to revise these competencies to reflect the maturity of palliative care and the evolution of primary palliative nursing. The result was *CARES: Competencies and Recommendations for Educating Under-graduate Nursing Students; Preparing Nurses to Care for the Seriously Ill and Their Families.*[44] In 2019, graduate nursing faculty developed competencies for graduate prepared nurses called *Graduate Competencies and Recommendations for Educating Nursing Students* (*G-CARES*).[45] These competencies are being integrated into professional nursing education on both the prelicensure (associate and bachelor's) and graduate (master's and doctoral) levels and were updated in 2022.

In addition, there was the development of two important curricula, one for nursing, the End-of-Life Nursing Education Consortium (ELNEC), and the other for physicians, Education for Physicians in End-of-Life Care (EPEC). Developed by expert palliative care nurse educators, the curriculum offers content and teaching resources to enhance palliative care competency. ELNEC, now in its twentieth year, has utilized a train-the-trainer model in which over forty thousand nurses and other health care professionals across all fifty US states and one hundred countries on six continents have participated in in-person training. These trainers have then provided education for one million nurses and other health care providers.[46] Its online course has been accessed by thousands of nurses. Over the years, there have been many versions, including core, graduate, oncology, critical care, geriatrics, pediatrics, veterans, advanced practice registered nurses, and doctor of nursing practice.[47]

Part 3 of the Strengthening Nursing Education to Improve End-of-Life Care Project was intended to support key organizations to improve end-of-life education for nursing. This resulted in the creation of the Nursing Leadership Consortium on End-of-Life Care. Funded by the Project on Death in America, its goal was to design a nursing agenda for end-of-life care.[48] This agenda emphasized educating nurse leaders in planning and managing change and advocacy in palliative and end-of-life care; developing systems that provided support; networking; providing mentorship for nurses engaged in advocacy and leadership in palliative and end-of-life care; and developing and implementing innovative strategies to further the Nursing Leadership Consortium priorities.[49]

ENSURING QUALITY PALLIATIVE CARE

Quality in palliative care has been a newer theme. When palliative care was first developed, it was based on the quality promoted by the Medicare Hospice Benefit.

However, that was not enough, and there was extreme variation in interpretation. I was a participant in the 2001 meeting to consider national standards in pallia- tive care. The group was wide and diverse. Over the next year, a working group was established. I was smitten with this work and ended up serving as the editor for the second and third editions of the Clinical Practice Guidelines for Quality Palliative Care, each time being thrilled at how they have been integrated into the field, representing practice outside the hospital in the community, and for the full lifespan ranging from neonates to octogenarians and beyond.

The next hurdle was offering quality palliative care. There was recognition that, while hospice quality and consistency were delineated within the federal Medi- care Hospice Benefit, there was nothing to delineate palliative care. The result was variation in how palliative care was being interpreted. To tackle this issue, in 2001, there was a meeting of interdisciplinary national leaders who repre- sented the field and various professional hospice and palliative organizations. The outcome was the creation of the National Consensus Project for Quality Palliative Care (NCP), a coalition of five organizations: Center to Advance Palliative Care (CAPC), American Academy of Hospice and Palliative Medi- cine (AAHPM), Hospice and Palliative Nurses Association (HPNA), National Hospice and Palliative Care Organization (NHPCO), and Last Acts.

The mission of the NCP was to create clinical practice guidelines to ensure consistency and quality of palliative care across the United States. The goal of the *Clinical Practice Guidelines for Quality Palliative Care* was (1) to promote quality and reduce variation in new and existing programs, (2) to develop and encourage continuity of care across settings, and (3) to facilitate collabora- tive partnerships among palliative care programs, community hospices, and a wide range of other health care delivery settings.[50] Interprofessional work group members representing all settings worked for three years on guidelines. More important, the document was achieved through a consensus process in which every line had 80 percent agreement. Finally, the document contained a first collection of evidence on palliative care published in the literature to support practice. The result was a 2004 publication that delineated eight domains of care, which remarkably have remained intact over three subse- quent editions, in 2009, 2013, and 2018:[51]

Domain 1: Structure and processes of care
Domain 2: Physical aspects of care

Domain 3: Psychological and psychiatric aspects of care

Domain 4: Social aspects of care

Domain 5: Spiritual, religious, and existential aspects of care

Domain 6: Cultural aspects of care

Domain 7: Care of the patient nearing the end of life (this title has changed twice)

Domain 8: Ethical and legal aspects of care [52]

These guidelines are a foundation to major palliative nursing initiatives: the HPNA Education *RN Education Design, HPNA Standards for Clinical Education*, the HPNA Oxford Manuals, and ground the modules of ELNEC.[53] These have also played an essential role in quality, as demonstrated by their adoption by the National Quality Forum for health care metrics.[54] They are playing a role in developing hospice and palliative RN and APRN residencies.

In 2006, the National Quality Forum created *A National Framework and Preferred Practices for Palliative and Hospice Care Quality: A Consensus Report*, which formulated palliative care standards and preferred practices by integrating these guidelines.[55] More importantly, they have been recognized by the Center for Medicare and Medicaid Services (CMS), with implications for reimbursement, internal and external quality measurement, regulation, and accreditation.[56] The NCP *Clinical Practice Guidelines* have served as the basis of palliative care program designation by the Joint Commission (TJC), DNV-GL Healthcare for hospital-based care; the Joint Commission, Accreditation Commission for Health Care (ACHC); and Community Health Accreditation Partners (CHAP) for community-based care.[57]

To continue the focus of palliative care across health care, various disciplines have partnered to develop quality measures. The American Academy of Hospice and Palliative Medicine and the Hospice and Palliative Nurses Association collaborated on *Measuring What Matters* to develop ten measures for hospice and palliative care.[58] Their aim is that measures should be concordant with the NCP *Clinical Practice Guidelines*, cut across various serious illnesses that should receive both primary and specialty palliative care, and be harmonious with work of the National Quality Forum.[59] The National Quality Forum created the Measurement Applications Partnership (MAP) with various work groups: clinician, hospital, and post-acute/long-term care. Various hospice and palliative nurses have served on these, including Dr. Carol

Spence, a nurse researcher at the National Hospice and Palliative Care Organization; Dr. Joy Goebel, a nurse researcher; and this author.

PALLIATIVE ADVANCED PRACTICE REGISTERED NURSE (APRN) DEVELOPMENT

In the late 1990s, there were only about ten nursing professionals practicing full-time palliative care. To have more ability to practice across settings and lead initiatives, I returned to school to obtain my education as an adult nurse practitioner. I collected contact information on file cards and created a listserv on the internet, which established a national network to support each other in practice issues and role delineation. Moreover, we shared experiences about program development and worked together to help our colleagues understand our broad scope of practice and reimbursement potential. In my case, it was clear I needed to develop a process to become a partner in weekend rounding to share the burden with physician colleagues. Since there was not a precedent for this at my organization, I met with the associate chief of nursing to create a structure for this. I built my structure from the midwives and the oncology nurse practitioners. Being the sole nurse practitioner working with seven palliative physicians necessitated frequent meetings for algorithms of care to ensure similar high-quality, evidence-based practice, while acknowledging our own art within patient care.

Another theme that arose in the development of the specialty of palliative nursing was the establishment of the palliative APRN. Within the Medicare Hospice Benefit, APRNs had to practice as RNs in hospice, because it did not recognize the different levels of nursing practice. This was an opportunity to develop the palliative APRN role. With the graying of America, it was recognized that APRNs would be necessary to work collaboratively with physicians in a variety of settings.

To promote consistency, nurse practitioners and clinical nurse specialists began to work on advanced competencies for assessing, prescribing, and managing patients with serious illnesses as well as being a full partner in palliative program development.[60] Specialty graduate education was led by Denice Sheehan, who developed a program for clinical nurse specialists at Ursuline College, and Deborah Witt Sherman, who led a nurse practitioner program at New York University.[61] A specialty advanced practice hospice and palliative examination was developed as a partnership between the American Nurses Credentialing Center (ANCC) and the National Board for Certification of Hospice and Palliative Nurses (NBCHPN). The exam was first offered in 2003; in 2007, the Centers for Medicare and Medicaid Services (CMS) recognized the APRN exam as a primary certification.[62] Moreover, the 2011 version of the Hospice Conditions of Participation allowed the hospice APRN to serve as attending provider for hospice patients and to provide face-to-face visits.[63]

In 2001, a summit of national nursing leaders representing clinical practice, academia, and research met in Pennsylvania. We spent the day reviewing the current environment, evidence of care, and the need for all clinicians to be all in for the impending gray tsunami. The result was *Advanced Practice Nurses Role in Palliative Care—A Position Statement from American Nursing Leaders,* which outlined the unique role of APRNs in palliative care.[64] The position statement acknowledged the APRN role in palliative care as a "valuable resource in national efforts to improve care and quality of life for Americans and their families living with advanced, life-limiting illness."[65] There were six recommendations that are just as pertinent today as in 2001.

1. PROFESSIONAL ASSOCIATIONS in nursing medicine, hospice and palliative care are called to engage in dialogue about the APN role and opportunities and strategies to advance it in palliative care.

2. NURSING EDUCATORS must become knowledgeable about palliative care, and
   - Develop continuing education to prepare existing APNs in palliative care competencies . . . ;
   - Integrate core palliative care competencies into the education of all APN students . . . ;
   - Develop clinical tracks for APN students who intend to specialize in palliative care.

3. PAYERS OF HEALTH SERVICES are called upon to recognize the specialty of palliative care and provide APNs with adequate and consistent compensation that is commensurate with APN scope of practice, authority and responsibility, regardless of practice setting. . . .

4. THE NATIONAL COUNCIL OF STATE BOARDS OF NURSING and individual state boards of nursing are called on to work collaboratively to

consistently recognize APN scopes of practice and privileges regardless of specialty and subspecialty.

5. HEALTH SYSTEMS OR HEALTH SERVICE PROVIDERS are asked to develop or expand practice opportunities for APNs in all settings that care for patients who may experience a life-limiting illness.

6. ADVANCED PRACTICE NURSES who practice in palliative care are called on to document and disseminate the outcome of their practice experience and roles, engage in interdisciplinary research, and translate research findings into practice.[66]

To ensure continued specialty APRN quality education, there has been work toward a consensus document for subspecialty palliative nursing content in master and doctor of nursing practice programs. To promote greater numbers of specialty palliative APRNs, there is increased interest in palliative APRN fellowships in both academic and community settings with guidelines for quality and consistent training, along with APRN mentors.

DEVELOPING THE EVIDENCE FOR PALLIATIVE CARE

When developing the NCP Clinical Practice Guidelines, there was a need to find the evidence to support the principles. I volunteered myself and Andy Billings to do this task, for which he never forgave me. We searched the literature for palliative care in the United States. It was a new specialty, and we found there was little specific to it in the American literature. Therefore, it was necessary to use literature about other specialties. In subsequent editions, I enlisted graduate students to assist in this work as part of their capstone projects. The evidence of palliative care continued to grow, across all settings and all populations and across diseases. The growth over twenty years is impressive, including the fact that the National Institutes of Health bases palliative care research in the National Institute of Nursing Research, as palliative care is a pillar of nursing practice.

With the development of guidelines and standards, it was necessary to develop evidence for the effectiveness of palliative care. In 2004, the first National Institutes of Health (NIH) State of the Science Conference on Improving End-of-Life Care was held in Bethesda. It was notably convened under the National Institute of Nursing Research, with a ten-member multidisciplinary planning committee consisting of four nurses, two physicians, two policy professors, one ethicist, and one researcher.[67] Chaired by Dr. Margaret Heitkemper, a professor at the University of Washington School of Nursing, the panel noted a lack of quality measures, a lack of communication, and the need for further research on palliative care delivery models, interventions, treatment, and outcomes. The conference further guided work to develop the evidence base for palliative care. A follow-up meeting, The Science of Compassion: Future Directions in End-of-Life and Palliative Care, was held in 2011. Again, organized under the National Institute of Nursing Research by an interdisciplinary panel, this conference had four goals.

- Examine the current status of palliative care and end-of-life research and practice
- Propose strategies to overcome barriers and ensure scientific/methodological rigor
- Delineate action items to galvanize progress in vital palliative research
- Envision and map ways to achieve a future rich with scientific endeavor and achievements[68]

Over the seven years between the two conferences, there had been a significant increase in palliative research, education, and translation into practice. Now there are even conferences solely devoted to the scientific aspects of palliative care, thus promoting further research. This bodes well for continued evolution of the field.

THE FUTURE OF PALLIATIVE CARE AND PALLIATIVE NURSING

As the field matures, the work to hone the field continues. In 2011, the Institute of Medicine released The Future of Nursing: Leading Change, Advancing Health, which had four points that are important to palliative nursing.

1. Nurses are vital to health care and reform, which is consistent in palliative care as nurses are needed to create new models for access to palliative care in underresourced areas.

2. Nurses can lead change as demonstrated by hospice care development in the United States under nursing leadership, including nursing leadership in the community.

3. Nurses should practice to the full extent of their education and license, compatible with the essential role palliative nurses play within palliative care as a whole.

4. Nurses should be encouraged to attain higher levels of education, which will help with palliative care capacity across all health settings.[69]

In 2021, the National Academy of Medicine followed up with the *Future of Nursing, 2020–2030: Charting a Path to Achieve Health Equity*. Again, the highlights are appropriate to palliative care because the palliative care literature has highlighted the health disparities that have existed in palliative care and that were magnified during the COVID-19 pandemic. With a long-standing role in public health, nursing has a role in leading and advancing health equity, particularly in the community, which is the next place for strategic development of palliative care. The report reemphasized lifting nursing practice barriers to increase access, which is pertinent to palliative care as there is much variability to palliative care practice by state and organization. It supported better payment models for nurses since they often address social determinants of care, which are a large part of palliative care delivery. It promoted the focus on developing nurse leaders, which is essential in palliative care when one looks at the paucity of attention to palliative nurse leaders over the years of palliative care. There is a focus on the well-being of nursing, which has always been a focus within palliative care due to the nature of the work. Finally, palliative nursing has been essential in the COVID-19 pandemic and other health crises caused by natural disasters or humanitarian crises. Palliative care and nursing have been an essential part of responding to these recent crises and should be involved in planning for future crises as well.

In 2014, the Institute of Medicine released *Dying in America: Improving Quality and Honoring Individual Preferences Near the End of Life*. The report identified five areas for quality palliative care in achieving health care improvement and moving care upstream to patients with serious illness, rather than focusing only on the end of life.

1. Delivery of person-centered and family-focused palliative care
2. Clinician-patient communication and advance care planning

3. Professional education in palliative care
4. Policies and payment for palliative care
5. Public education and engagement in palliative care

This document has provided a road map for further work in palliative care.

I have worked to translate seminal documents to reflect nursing. I continue to work on models of education for the next generation and fostering nursing leadership. I was a coeditor of the 2014 Advancing Expert Care *Palliative Nursing Leadership Position Statement*.[70] I also participated in the Palliative and End-of-Life Nursing Panel that developed the *Call to Action—Nurses Lead and Transform Palliative Care*.[71] This is a blueprint specific to nursing articulated by the American Nurses Association and the Hospice and Palliative Nurses Association, which states that, because all nurses practice palliative care, they need skill development in communication, particularly since communication for registered nurses is predicated on scope of practice.[72] Among the key messages are the adoption of the End of Life Nurse Education Consortium (ELNEC) Curriculum as fundamental education; the use of the NCP *Clinical Practice Guidelines* to promote the specialty; the development of new models of care, particularly in the community; and the presence of nursing on health care, regulatory, and other decision-making bodies.[73]

To achieve these goals, leadership will be necessary. For example, the Cambia Health Foundation has created a Sojourns Leadership Program for palliative care providers.[74] Each year since 2014, ten to twelve palliative care professionals have been chosen as Sojourns Scholars. As of 2021, eighteen of seventy-four scholars are nurses.[75] All of the Sojourns Scholars are initiating a variety of educational and research initiatives to further the field. Their projects span all aspects of palliative care, including program development, technology to improve the patient experience, communication that is inclusive to all cultures, and health equity to ensure access to quality care across populations.[76]

CONCLUSION

The foundation of modern nursing was built upon caring for individuals with life-limiting diseases and conditions. Palliative care is synergistic with the foundations of nursing, given its focus on supporting care of patients with serious illness. Since the principles of nursing and palliative care are so closely aligned, nursing has an essential role in palliative care. It may be that without this nursing presence, hospice and palliative care might not have developed in the way it did. Given their close proximity to patients and the fact they spend the most amount of time at the bedside with them, nurses will continue to refine the art and science of primary and specialty palliative nursing. However, further maturation necessitates continued interdisciplinary collaboration, recognizing the unique role of each discipline in helping create innovative models of care delivery, particularly in the community and within vulnerable populations to ensure health equity and reduce the influence of structural racism.

Palliative nursing in the United States has had a rich and illustrious role in the evolution of both hospice and palliative care. The outlook of palliative care for the future is bright, with possibilities and innovation still to come from the next generation of nurses and their interprofessional partners.

NOTES

1. World Health Organization 2020.
2. Ibid.
3. Craven and Wald 1975; Buck 2006.
4. Amenta and Bohnet 1975.
5. Ibid.; Buck 2006.
6. Farren 2003.
7. Dahlin 2010.
8. Buck 2006; Campbell 1986.
9. Farren 2003.
10. Buck 2006.
11. Saunders 1999.
12. Saunders 2001, v.
13. Buck 2006.
14. Kübler-Ross 1969.
15. Yale Bulletin 2001.
16. Ibid.
17. Ibid.
18. US Department of Health and Human Services et al. 1981.
19. Ibid.
20. Foster and Corless 1999, 12.
21. Dahlin 2021.
22. American Nurses Association 1987.
23. Ibid.
24. Dahlin 2021.
25. Ibid.
26. Dahlin, Coyne, et al. 2019.
27. Dahlin 1999, 75–84.
28. Robert Wood Johnson Foundation and Milbank Memorial Fund 2000.
29. Open Society Institute 1998, 2001, 2003.
30. Robert Wood Johnson Foundation and Milbank Memorial Fund 2000.
31. Promoting Excellence in End of Life Care 2002b.
32. Solomon et al. 1993.
33. SUPPORT Principal Investigators 1995.
34. Institute of Medicine 1997.
35. Ibid.
36. Institute of Medicine 2002.
37. Last Acts 2002.
38. American Nurses Association 2021; National Academy of Sciences, Engineering and Medicine 2021.
39. Ferrell, Grant, and Virani 1999; Last Acts 2001, 2002; Dahlin and Mazanec 2011.
40. Weisfeld et al. 2000.
41. Ferrell, Grant, and Virani 1999.
42. Wendt 2001.
43. American Association of Colleges of Nursing 1997.
44. American Association of Colleges of Nursing 2016.

45. American Association of Colleges of Nursing 2019.

46. "About ELNEC" n.d.

47. Ibid.

48. Dahlin and Mazanec 2011.

49. Ibid.

50. National Consensus Project for Quality Palliative Care 2004.

51. National Consensus Project for Quality Palliative Care 2004, 2009, 2013, 2018.

52. National Consensus Project for Quality Palliative Care 2018.

53. "About ELNEC" n.d.; Dahlin 2016; Hospice and Palliative Nurses Association 2015; HPNA Palliative Nursing Manuals 2019.

54. National Quality Forum 2006; National Quality Forum 2016.

55. National Quality Forum 2006.

56. Ibid.; National Quality Forum 2016.

57. Joint Commission n.d., "Palliative Care Certification"; DNV GL Healthcare 2018; Accreditation Commission for Health Care 2018; Community Health Accreditation Program 2018; Joint Commission n.d., "Certification Options."

58. American Academy of Hospice and Palliative Medicine 2019.

59. Ibid.

60. Hospice and Palliative Nurses Association 2002.

61. Promoting Excellence in End of Life Care 2002a.

62. Dahlin 2021.

63. Department of Health and Human Services and Centers for Medicare and Medicaid Services 2011.

64. Promoting Excellence in End of Life Care 2002a.

65. Ibid.

66. Ibid.

67. National Institutes of Health 2004.

68. National Institute of Nursing Research 2011.

69. Institute of Medicine 2011.

70. Hospice and Palliative Nurses Association, Hospice and Palliative Credentialing Center, and Hospice and Palliative Nurses Foundation 2014.

71. American Nurses Association Professional Issues Panel 2017.

72. Ibid.

73. Ibid.

74. Cambia Health Foundation 2021.

75. Ibid.

76. Kamal et al. 2016; Cruz-Oliver et al. 2017; Dahlin, Sanders, et al. 2019.

WORKS CITED

"About ELNEC." n.d. American Association of Colleges of Nursing. Accessed June 19, 2021. https://www.aacnnursing.org/ELNEC/About.

Accreditation Commission for Health Care. 2022. "Palliative Care Accreditation." Accessed May 24, 2022. https://www.achc.org/palliative-care.

Amenta, M., and N. Bohnet. 1986. *Nursing Care of the Terminally Ill.* Boston: Little, Brown.

American Academy of Hospice and Palliative Medicine. 2019. "Measuring What Matters." Accessed June 19, 2021. http://aahpm.org/uploads/education/MWM%20FAQ%20List.pdf.

American Association of Colleges of Nursing. 1997. "Peaceful Death: Recommended Competencies and Curricular Guidelines for End-of-Life Nursing Care." Washington, DC: AACN.

Accessed June 19, 2021. https://eric.ed.gov/?id=ED453706.

———. 2016. "CARES: Competencies and Recommendations for Educating Undergraduate Nursing Students: Preparing Nurses to Care for the Seriously Ill and Their Families." Washington, DC: AACN. Accessed June 19, 2021. https://www.aacnnursing.org/Portals/42/ELNEC/PDF/New-Palliative-Care-Competencies.pdf.

———. 2019. "Preparing Graduate Nursing Students to Ensure Quality Palliative Care for the Seriously Ill and Their Families." Washington, DC: AACN. Accessed June 19, 2021. https://www.aacnnursing.org/Portals/42/ELNEC/PDF/Graduate-CARES.pdf.

American Nurses Association. 1987. *Standards and Scope of Hospice Nursing Practice.*

Kansas City, MO: American Nurses Association.

American Nurses Association Professional Issues Panel. 2017. "A Call for Action—Nurses Lead and Transform Palliative Care." American Nurses Association. Accessed June 19, 2021. http://www.nursingworld.org/CallforAction-NursesLeadTransformPalliativeCare.

Buck, J. 2006. "Reweaving a Tapestry of Care: Religion, Nursing, and the Meaning of Hospice, 1945–1978." Nursing History Review 15:113–45.

Cambia Health Foundation. 2019. Sojourns Scholar Leadership Program. Portland, OR: CHF. June 19, 2021. https://www.cambiahealthfoundation.org/funding-areas/sojourns-scholars-leadership-program.html.

Campbell, L. 1986. "History of the Hospice Movement." Cancer Nursing 9 (6): 333–38.

Community Health Accreditation Program. 2018. Palliative Care Guidelines. Washington, DC: CHAP. Accessed June 19, 2021. https://education.chaplinq.org/products/chap-palliative-care-certification-standards.

Craven, J., and F. Wald. 1975. "Hospice Care for Dying Patients." American Journal of Nursing 75:1816–22.

Cruz-Oliver, D. M., R. Bernacki, Z. Cooper, C. Grudzen, S. Izumi, D. Lafond, D. Lam, T. W. LeBlanc, J. Tjia, and J. Walter. 2017. "The Cambia Sojourns Scholars Leadership Program: Conversations with Emerging Leaders in Palliative Care." Journal of Palliative Medicine 20 (8): 804–12.

Dahlin, C. 1999. "Access to Care." Hospice Journal 14 (3–4):75–84.

———. 2010. "Communication in Palliative Care: An Essential Competency for Nurses." In Oxford Textbook of Palliative Nursing, 3rd ed., edited by B. R. Ferrell and N. Coyle, 107–33. New York: Oxford University Press.

———. 2016. RN Education Design. Pittsburgh: Hospice and Palliative Nurses Association.

———. 2021. Palliative Nursing: Scope and Standards of Practice. 6th ed. Pittsburgh:

Hospice and Palliative Nurses Association.

Dahlin, C., P. Coyne, J. Goldberg, and L. Vaughn. 2019. "Palliative Care Leadership." Journal of Palliative Care 34 (1): 21–28.

Dahlin, C., and P. Mazanec. 2011. "Building from Our Past: Celebrating 25 Years of Clinical Practice in Hospice and Palliative Nursing." Journal of Hospice and Palliative Nursing 13 (6): S20–S28.

Dahlin, C., J. Sanders, B. Calton, S. DeSanto-Madeya, D. Donesky, J. R. Lakin, E. Roeland, J. S. Scherer, A. Walling, and B. Williams. 2019. "The Cambia Sojourns Scholars Leadership Program: Projects and Reflections on Leadership in Palliative Care." Journal of Palliative Medicine 22 (7): 823–29.

Department of Health and Human Services and Centers for Medicare and Medicaid Services. 2011. "CMS Manual System: Pub 100-02 Medicare Benefit Policy: Transmittal 141." Accessed June 19, 2021. https://www.cms.gov/Regulations-and-Guidance/Guidance/Transmittals/downloads/R141BP.pdf.

DNV GL Healthcare. 2018. Healthcare Palliative Program Certification Requirements. Milford, OH: DNV GL Healthcare. Accessed June 19, 2021. https://www.dnvgl.us/assurance/healthcare/PalliativeCare.html.

Farren, S. 2003. "The Sister Nurses." Health Progress (March–April 2003). Accessed June 19, 2021. https://www.chausa.org/docs/default-source/health-progress/the-sister-nurses-pdf.pdf?sfvrsn=2.

Ferrell, B. R., M. Grant, and R. Virani. 1999. "Strengthening Nursing Education to Improve End-of-Life Care." Nursing Outlook 47 (6): 252–56.

Foster, Z., and I. B. Corless. 1999. "Origins: An American Perspective." Hospice Journal 14 (3–4): 9–13.

Hospice and Palliative Nurses Association. 2002. Competencies for the Hospice and Palliative APN. Pittsburgh: HPNA.

———. 2015. HPNA Standards for Clinical Education of Hospice and Palliative Nurses. Pittsburgh: HPNA.

HPNA Palliative Nursing Manuals. 2019. New York: Oxford University Press.

Institute of Medicine. 1997. *Approaching Death: Improving Care at the End of Life.* Washington, DC: National Academies Press.

———. 2002. *When Children Die: Improving Palliative and End-of-Life Care for Children and Their Families.* Washington, DC: National Academies Press.

———. 2011. *The Future of Nursing: Leading Change, Advancing Health.* Washington, DC: National Academies Press.

———. 2014. *Dying in America: Improving Quality and Honoring Individual Preferences Near End of Life.* Washington, DC: National Academies Press.

Joint Commission. n.d. "Certification Options." Accessed May 24, 2022. https://www .jointcommission.org/accreditation-and -certification/health-care-settings/home -care/excel/certification-options.

———. n.d. "Palliative Care Certification." Accessed May 24, 2022. https://www .jointcommission.org/accreditation-and -certification/certification/certifications -by-setting/hospital-certifications /palliative-care-certification.

Kamal, A. H., W. G. Anderson, R. D. Boss, A. A. Brody, T. C. Campbell, C. J. Creutzfeldt, C. J. Hurd, A. L. Kinderman, E. C. Lindenberger, and L. F. Reinke. 2016. "The Cambia Sojourns Scholars Leadership Program: Project Summaries from the Inaugural Scholar Cohort." *Journal of Palliative Medicine* 19 (6): 591–600.

Kübler-Ross, E. 1969. *On Death and Dying.* New York: Macmillan.

Last Acts. 2001. *Transforming Death in America.* Washington, DC: Last Acts.

———. 2002. *Means to a Better End: A Report on Dying in America Today.* Washington, DC: Last Acts.

National Academies of Sciences, Engineering, and Medicine. 2021. *The Future of Nursing, 2020–2030: Charting a Path to Achieve Health Equity.* Washington, DC: National Academies Press.

National Consensus Project for Quality Palliative Care. 2004. *Clinical Practice Guidelines for Quality Palliative Care.* Pittsburgh: National Consensus Project for Quality Palliative Care.

———. 2009. *Clinical Practice Guidelines for Quality Palliative Care.* 2nd ed. Pittsburgh: National Consensus Project.

———. 2013. *Clinical Practice Guidelines for Quality Palliative Care.* 3rd ed. Pittsburgh: National Consensus Project for Quality Palliative Care.

———. 2018. *Clinical Practice Guidelines for Quality Palliative Care.* 4th ed. Richmond, VA: National Hospice and Palliative Care Coalition. https://www .nationalcoalitionhpc.org/ncp.

National Institute of Nursing Research. 2011. "The Science of Compassion: Future Directions in End-of-Life and Palliative Care." Accessed May 23, 2022. https:// www.ninr.nih.gov/sites/files/docs /science-of-compassion-executive -summary.pdf.

National Institutes of Health. 2004. "NIH State-of-the-Science Conference Statement on Improving End-of-Life Care." *NIH Consensus and State-of-the-Science Statements* 21 (3): 1–26.

National Quality Forum. 2006. *A National Framework and Preferred Practices for Palliative and Hospice Care Quality: A Consensus Report.* Washington, DC: NQF.

———. 2016. *Palliative Care and End-of-Life Care.* Washington, DC: NQF. Accessed June 19, 2021. http://www.qualityforum .org/Topics/Palliative_Care_and_End -of-Life_Care.aspx.

Open Society Institute. 1998. *Project on Death in America.* New York: Project on Death in America.

———. 2001. *Project on Death in America—January 1998–December 2000.* New York: Project on Death in America.

———. 2003. *Project on Death in America—January 2001–December 2003 Report of Activities.* New York: Project on Death in America.

Promoting Excellence in End of Life. 2002a. *Advanced Practice Nurses Role in Palliative Care: A Position Statement from American Nursing Leaders.* Missoula, MT: Promoting Excellence. Accessed June 19, 2021. https://www.promoting

excellence.org/downloads/apn
_position.pdf.

———. 2002b. *Advanced Practice Nursing: Pioneering Practices in Palliative Care.* Missoula, MT: Promoting Excellence. Accessed June 19, 2021. https://www .promotingexcellence.org/downloads /apn_report.pdf.

The Robert Wood Johnson Foundation and Milbank Memorial Fund. 2000. *Pioneer Programs in Palliative Care: Nine Case Studies.* New York: Milbank Memorial Fund.

Saunders, D. C. 1999. "Origins: International Perspectives, Then and Now." *Hospice Journal* 14 (3–4): 1–7.

———. 2001. Foreword to *Oxford Textbook of Palliative Nursing,* edited by B. R. Ferrell and N. Coyle. New York: Oxford University Press.

Solomon, M. Z., L. O'Donnell, B. Jennings, V. Guilfoy, S. M. Wolf, K. Nolan, R. Jackson, D. Koch-Weser, and S. Donnelley. 1993. "Decisions Near the End of Life: Professional Views on Life-Sustaining Treatments." *American Journal of Public Health* 83 (1): 14–23.

SUPPORT Principal Investigators. 1995. "A Controlled Trial to Improve Care for the Seriously Ill Hospitalized Patients: The Study to Understand Prognoses and Preferences for Outcomes and Risks of Treatments (SUPPORT)." *JAMA* 274 (20): 1591–98.

US Department of Health and Human Services, Public Health Service, Health Resources Administration, Bureau of Health Professions, Division of Nursing. 1981. *Hospice Education Program for Nurses.* Hyattsville, MD: Health Resources Administration.

Weisfeld, V., D. Miller, R. Gibson, and S. Schroeder. 2000. "Improving Care at the End of Life: What Does It Take?" *Health Affairs* 19 (6): 277–83.

Wendt, A. 2001. "End-of-Life Competencies and the NCLEX-RN Examination." *Nursing Outlook* 49 (3): 138–41.

World Health Organization. 2020. "Palliative Care." August 5, 2020. Accessed May 23, 2022. https://www.who.int/news-room /fact-sheets/detail/palliative-care.

Yale Bulletin. "American Academy Honors Three from YSN." 2001. New Haven: Yale University. Accessed June 19, 2021. http://archives.news.yale.edu/v30.n11 /story9.html.

CHAPTER 2

The Challenge of Bringing Palliative Medicine and Person-Centered Care to Large Hospitals and Universities

Eduardo Bruera

I met a sixty-year-old man with metastatic lung cancer who had been referred to the Supportive Care Center by his oncologist because of increasing chest pain. Our team's assessment showed that the patient had not only pain but also fatigue, anorexia, weight loss, depression, anxiety, and significant family distress. Our assessment showed that some of the physical and emotional symptoms of the patient were not only due to his advanced cancer and the side effects of the chemotherapy and immunotherapy he was receiving; the symptoms were also a result of having significant relationship problems with his wife, losing his job due to his illness, and being unable to face many of the financial pressures associated with paying multiple bills and living expenses. Our plan of care included significant changes in his opioid analgesics, medications for the management of anorexia, and help for the prevention of constipation, nausea, and fatigue, as well as counseling for the patient and his wife and discussions regarding financial support. At the follow-up visit two weeks later, the patient expressed a significant reduction in his overall symptom distress.

As this story illustrates, the diagnosis of cancer and other serious illnesses is associated with multiple physical symptoms such as pain, fatigue, shortness of breath, lack of appetite, and inability to sleep.[1] Patients also experience emotional distress, including anxiety and depression.[2] Finally, serious illness and its treatment impact the patient's ability to function and relate to family and friends, the patient's spiritual experience, and the present and future financial health of patient and family alike. Suffering, in short, is both a multidimensional experience of those who become seriously ill and a near-universal experience as well, even among those whose disease can be successfully cured or controlled for a long period of time.[3]

Given this well-known fact, it would be reasonable to expect that major hospitals and outpatient care facilities should devote a considerable proportion of their resources to the appropriate diagnosis and alleviation of suffering, perhaps by offering educational opportunities. It would be reasonable, too, to imagine that universities would have major research efforts devoted to how to manage physical and emotional suffering among patients and their loved ones.

Unfortunately, this is not the case. Health care institutions, both academic and nonacademic, follow a strong biomedical model. They are largely organized to deliver impeccable clinical care, research, and education related to specific diseases but often poorly prepared to address and alleviate multidimensional suffering.

There have been major developments in the diagnosis and the treatment of many diseases, and, when new knowledge appears, it is rapidly implemented and adopted, making it accessible to patients. Yet new interventions to alleviate pain, shortness of breath, fatigue, depression and anxiety, emotional distress, and spiritual suffering have been much slower to develop. Consequently, such interventions are, by and large, inaccessible to patients and their loved ones.

We cannot solve all the issues of total pain, nor can we alleviate every sort of suffering. But we *can* identify some of the most common challenges to alleviating total pain, and we can imagine possible ways to address it. That, in the end, is the challenge posed to those of us who are committed to implementing supportive palliative care in academic centers.

UNITED KINGDOM HOSPICE MOVEMENT

During the 1960s, in response to situations such as this one, a small group of physicians, nurses, and other health care professionals had already become alarmed by the almost universal domination of biomedical aspects in health care institutions and medical schools.[4] The alleviation of physical, psychosocial, and spiritual distress had become progressively less important; the overwhelming majority of medical schools and hospitals lacked structures, processes, and outcomes to address patient and family suffering.

This small group of hospice pioneers understood that suffering is at its most intense close to the end of life. They decided to offer care to patients at the end of life in residential hospices in the community. These inpatient facilities provided close attention to physical, psychosocial, and spiritual distress. They implemented an approach characterized by interdisciplinary teams under the leadership of the first generation of hospice physicians. What was initially a local and limited phenomenon in scattered areas of the United Kingdom rapidly became global, as groups of health care professionals in other countries in the developed and developing world perceived similar needs for their patients.[5]

The vast majority of funding for the initial hospices in the United Kingdom came from community donations. Local neighborhoods contributed to the maintenance of hospice organizations. Yet they were not the only ones to sacrifice for the cause, the promise of hospice care: the participating health care professionals received lesser reimbursement and had lower career expectations compared to those studying more traditional biomedical aspects of health care.

One of the main limitations of the original hospice movement in the United Kingdom was that these pioneer health care professionals had almost no access to patients in acute care, outpatient, or home care settings. Consequently, although this movement had a vast impact—it inspired the next generation of palliative care programs—a relative handful of physicians provided care to a small percentage of patients for a very short period of time, near the end of life.

Further, despite these early developments, the conditions for many patients did not improve. In 1979, for example, I saw a thirty-six-year-old patient with metastatic breast cancer when I was part of the oncology team in a major academic hospital. The patient had severe pain due to metastatic bone disease, and she was receiving intermittent intramuscular injections of meperidine as needed when the pain became very severe. She stated that she received minimal relief, and also had significant pain, after each injection. She also had significant fatigue, which made it difficult for her to communicate and take care of her two young children. At the time, there was no measurement of patient-reported outcomes. Even though the cancer was considered clearly incurable and progressive, she had not been informed of her disseminated disease and poor prognosis; she was given a minimum dosage of chemotherapy until she died in the hospital without receiving the visit of her children and extended family.

THE EMERGENCE OF PALLIATIVE CARE

By the late 1970s and early 1980s, patients with advanced cancer and other incurable progressive diseases were frequently discharged to an inpatient hospice that was located closer to the patient's home. In these settings, patients received compassionate interdisciplinary care until the end of their lives. Unfortunately, this type of care was completely unavailable earlier in the trajectory of illness, including at all academic institutions and cancer centers. This resulted in patients experiencing a high level of suffering early in the trajectory of their illness while they were still receiving treatment that was beginning to be ineffective, with no access to significant physical, psychosocial, and spiritual support.

In the late 1970s and early 1980s, a group of physicians brought the principles of the hospice movement from Britain to North America. These programs started initially in Canada, where Dr. Balfour Mount coined the term "palliative care." Initial palliative care programs operated palliative care units in acute care hospitals, first in Canada and later around the world.[6] These palliative care units allowed patients who were not eligible for home hospice to access sophisticated care close to the end of their lives, under the able direction of interdisciplinary teams.

Since palliative care teams were now located within acute care facilities, they were able to extend their care to consultation for patients admitted to many other units in the hospital. The presence of palliative care teams in academic hospitals such as MD Anderson also afforded the opportunity to provide clinical research and teaching in multiple domains of palliative care.[7]

In the United States, in 1983, the Medicare Hospice Benefit was established. For patients with an expected survival of fewer than six months, Medicare would cover home hospice and some inpatient hospice care, as long as the patient agreed to forgo disease-directed therapy. This benefit promoted many hospice organizations across the United States, providing hospice access to a growing number of patients.

In the early 1990s, it became clear that the body of knowledge required to deliver hospice and palliative care was complex and that patient care would benefit from the establishment of a subspecialty. Initially in the United Kingdom, and later in most developed and developing countries, hospice and palliative medicine became a recognized subspecialty.[8] In 1987, in fact, the Royal College of Physicians of the United Kingdom recognized palliative medicine as a specialty certificate.

INTEGRATION OF EARLY PALLIATIVE AND SUPPORTIVE CARE

The impact of the hospice movement in the United Kingdom and early hospital-based palliative care was limited, as patients were only able to access services very late in the trajectory of their disease. In response, a number of pioneering outpatient programs attempted to deal with this late-referral phenomenon by offering services to ambulatory patients with serious illnesses and multidimensional suffering.[9] Since 2010, it has become apparent that providing patients early access to palliative care not only improved physical, psychosocial, spiritual, and family distress; it also improved financial outcomes.[10] These findings further encouraged palliative care expansion.

Another factor encouraging that expansion was a simple name change. Since the term "palliative care" was frequently associated with hospice and end-of-life care, many patients and referring physicians struggled with early referral, even though the benefits of early referral were clear. Some programs chose to change the name of their service from "palliative care" to "supportive care" or "supportive palliative care," with the latter term incorporated into Texas law in 2018. This simple name change has encouraged more frequent referrals at earlier stages of the disease trajectory.

CHANGING THE CULTURE

On any given day, every hospital has numerous patients experiencing severe multidimensional suffering. These hospitals have expensive intensive care units, interventional radiology suites, surgical robots, and emergency departments, yet most of them lack palliative care units—and many lack even a comprehensive supportive palliative care team to help treat the suffering!

Universities, granting agencies, and philanthropies have funded research for years, leading to multiple diagnostic and therapeutic improvements in cancer and other serious illness care. However, basic cancer and other serious illness symptom management is woefully antiquated on no fewer than two counts. First, it still begins with the Edmonton Symptom Assessment Scale, a nearly thirty-year-old numeric severity scale. Second, basic serious pain management continues to rely on drugs ranging from steroids to neuroleptics to opioids—drugs that are decades to hundreds of years old. Even though they are suboptimal, these medications can bring great relief to the distressing symptoms experienced by many patients; unfortunately, clinicians frequently underprescribe, or do not prescribe, these medications to patients in many hospitals.

Why do we see such a lack of progress? Several years ago, I proposed that the main barriers for both adult[11] and pediatric medicine are largely *cultural*.[12] During the last forty years of my professional life, medicine has focused upon biomedical issues. Much of medical training is based on an organ system and disease system approach. Palliative care is neither organ-centered nor disease-centered. Palliative care is person-centered care for the patient and family facing any serious illness. Embracing such a nonorgan system, nondisease system, person-centered approach is emotionally risky and has even been career-threatening to those who have promulgated this needed cultural change.[13] Fostering cultural change requires educating the very leaders who have excelled in the organ-system, disease-centered approach of most contemporary medicine. Fostering cultural change means providing compelling and convincing rationales to practitioners who feel threatened by a change in culture from an organ- and disease-centered approach to a nonorgan system, nondisease system, person-centered approach.

Not all leaders and institutions are able to make progress along the cultural pathway toward a palliative culture. There are four distinct stages in the adoption of a palliative culture. Each stage poses challenges.

1. Denial: At this stage, both individuals and organizations perceive no need for palliative care. The claim is that, both from a clinical and academic perspective, there is no need for this type of care and this body of knowledge. Unfortunately, at this stage of cultural change, individuals and institutions

are unlikely to provide funding for clinical or academic programs in palliative care. One way to address denial is to measure, in very simple ways (i.e., through surveys), the level of physical, emotional, social, spiritual, and financial distress of patients cared for in the institution. Data obtained can then help leaders move from denial to the next stage.

2. Palliphobia: At this stage, individuals and organizations become fearful of the potential negative consequences of developing palliative care. Many erroneously believe that palliative care will be misperceived as hospice, will discourage patients from coming to the hospital, and will result in financial losses. There is also the fear that supportive palliative care will signal failure—failure to heal all diseases. One may quote the literature refuting palliphobia, but just as much as all politics is local, so too is all health care. To counteract palliphobia, it is beneficial to create a database of success, which carefully measures patient improvement, especially among patients referred early to palliative care services. Once these data become available, it will be possible to present the results to the rest of the medical community in various institutions; this will promote a dialogue with the initial pioneers who referred patients to supportive palliative care.

3. Pallilalia: This is unfortunately the most dangerous stage in the development of a palliative care culture. Institutions and individuals frequently talk about the importance of palliative care but fail to provide palliative care teams with the resources they need to complete their work. In this stage, a supportive palliative care team is frequently flooded by consults and demands for care, without any of the major investments necessary to create processes of care and without adequate hiring of enough palliative care professionals to meet the evolving demand. Many palliative care teams collapse at this stage, burned out by increasing demands and static resources. It is important, therefore, to measure carefully the workload faced by palliative care teams and to compare it with a workload faced by other medical specialties in the same institution in order to ensure that the level of support is similar to the one existing for other specialties.

4. Palliactive: This final stage of development of a palliative culture can be identified by appropriate resources for clinical and academic work (if this care takes place in an academic center). Resources at this stage are based upon a safe administrative structure that provides not only appropriate benchmarks for productivity, but appropriate protections for the palliative care professionals involved in this challenging branch of medicine.

CONCLUSIONS

Is the glass of palliative care half empty or half full? On my pessimistic days, it seems to me that the pace of the adoption of supportive palliative care has been glacial. Major research and education needs have been identified, but the resources to meet those needs have yet to be adequately provided in most teaching institutions. We know that most medical care is provided outside of academic medical institutions, and relatively few of those institutions provide comprehensive, multidisciplinary, board-certified teams to treat the multidimensional suffering that exists in almost every hospital. One reason for this—and it is a reason that keeps me up at night—is that in the United States we graduate only about 350 palliative care specialists a year—not nearly enough for a country of 330 million persons, almost all of whom will someday benefit from palliative care services if they can find them.

On my more optimistic days, I recognize the growing number of papers published in multiple peer-reviewed academic journals that did not exist when I embarked on my professional journey. In addition, the National Quality Forum, the American Society of Clinical Oncology, and several other organizations have established standards for palliative care. I can also recall a time when one could count the number of palliative care programs in the United States on one hand; now there are a few thousand. On these optimistic days, I think that just maybe we are reaching a critical mass of health care professionals and leaders fully committed to the cultural change needed to provide true person-centered care.

NOTES

1. Hui and Bruera 2017.
2. Bruera 2019.
3. Cassell 2013.
4. Clark 2016, 59–84.
5. Ibid., 149–95.
6. Bruera and Pereira 1999.
7. Ibid.; Hui and Bruera 2016.
8. Bruera and Pereira 1999.
9. Hui et al. 2018.
10. Dalal and Bruera 2017.
11. Bruera 2004.
12. Friedrichsdorf and Bruera 2018.
13. Kamal et al. 2017, 2020.

WORKS CITED

Bruera, E. 2004. "The Development of a Palliative Care Culture." *Journal of Palliative Care* 20 (4): 316–19.

———. 2019. "Relieving Physical and Psychosocial Pain in Patients with Cancer—The Search for Enlightened

Academic Medical Leaders." *JAMA Oncology* 5 (10): 1401–2.

Bruera, E., and J. Pereira. 1999. "The Research Palliative Care Unit." *Cancer Treatment and Research* 100:161–83.

Cassell, E. J. 2013. "Sickness." In *The Nature of Healing*, 1–24. New York: Oxford University Press.

Clark, D. 2016. *To Comfort Always*. New York: Oxford University Press.

Dalal, S., and E. Bruera. 2017. "End-of-Life Care Matters: Palliative Cancer Care Results in Better Care and Lower Costs." *Oncologist* 22 (4): 361–68.

Friedrichsdorf, S. J., and E. Bruera. 2018. "Delivering Pediatric Palliative Care: From Denial, Palliphobia, Pallilalia to Palliactive." *Children (Basel)* 5 (9): 120–32.

Hui, D., and E. Bruera. 2016. "Integrating Palliative Care into the Trajectory of Cancer Care." *Nature Reviews Clinical Oncology* 13 (3): 159–71.

———. 2017. "The Edmonton Symptom Assessment System 25 Years Later: Past, Present, and Future Developments." *Journal of Pain and Symptom Management* 53 (3): 630–43.

Hui, D., B. L. Hannon, C. Zimmermann, and E. Bruera. 2018. "Improving Patient and Caregiver Outcomes in Oncology: Team-Based, Timely, and Targeted Palliative Care." *CA: A Cancer Journal for Clinicians* 68 (5): 356–76.

Kamal, A. H., J. H. Bull, K. M. Swetz, S. P. Wolf, T. D. Shanafelt, and E. R. Myers. 2017. "Future of the Palliative Care Workforce: Preview to an Impending Crisis." *American Journal of Medicine* 130 (2): 113–14.

Kamal, A. H., J. H. Bull, S. P. Wolf, K. M. Swetz, T. D. Shanafelt, K. Ast, D. Kavalieratos, and C. T. Sinclair. 2019. "Prevalence and Predictors of Burnout Among Hospice and Palliative Care Clinicians in the U.S." *Journal of Pain and Symptom Management* 59 (5): e6–e13.

CHAPTER 3

The Evolutionary Relationship of Oncology and Palliative Care

A Personal Journey

Neil MacDonald

I am a man of a certain age who has worked across the spectrum of cancer research and care for fifty-six years, dating from my training in medical oncology in 1962 at Memorial Sloan Kettering Cancer Center under the mentorship of the pioneering oncologist Dr. David Karnofsky—a very fine man who died too young.

Considering the reasons for which the editors asked me to write and the lived history I have to share, I will concentrate on how oncologists' appreciation of the psychosocial and spiritual aspects important to cancer patients and their families has changed over fifty-plus years. Much of this change encompasses the history of palliative care. I will consider these changes through the spectrum of cancer as this is my experience. Yet I am conscious that what I have to say applies to the care of patients with other life-threatening diseases.

1960s

Let's start in the 1960s. It was the era of "kill-the-tumor," even though, for patients with advanced solid cancer, cure was not an option (with the exception of choriocarcinoma, a rare malignancy). Young oncologists were taught to focus laser-like on the tumor, and success was simply measured by change in tumor mass and length of survival. The concept of palliative care was not on anyone's mind until 1967.

That year, a singular event happened: the first purpose-built modern hospice, St. Christopher's, was started by Dame Cicely Saunders in London, England. Dame Cicely was a remarkable woman. She had first trained as a nurse, then became a social worker and ultimately a physician—what a background for palliative care! During and after her medical training she worked at St. Joseph's Hospice, a hospice organized by an order of nuns. She started important research on pain management with opioids, acquired a special sensitivity to the dying, and developed the concept of "total pain." She realized suffering was not just physical but psychological, social, and spiritual as well.

1970S

My interest in palliative care was first awakened when I listened to a passionate, well-reasoned presentation about palliative care by a young urologic oncology surgeon from McGill, Balfour Mount. I once asked Bal how he became so passionate about the subject. He told me he was inspired by a lecture given by Dr. Elisabeth Kübler-Ross—of the "five stages of dying" fame. He then read her book *On Death and Dying* and noted many references to Cicely Saunders.

Bal gave Dame Saunders a cold call one morning and ended up with an invitation to work at St. Christopher's for one week. Within that short time, he was gobsmacked—absolutely moved by their work and their ability to control symptoms in an atmosphere of patient/staff partnership, providing superb clinical care established on a spiritual foundation. He returned to the Royal Victoria Hospital, McGill's great teaching hospital, where he conducted studies on the care of advanced cancer patients. The results were stunning. In this world-famous hospital, people were suffering terribly. The care provided was well-meaning but uninformed. This story was not unique to McGill. Indeed, palliative care owes much of its *raison d'être* to the revelation that our cancer centers and hospitals, great and small, were derelict in the care of their suffering and dying patients. That made Bal different; he decided to do something about it.

Bal started the McGill Palliative Care Program in 1974, introducing the phrase "palliative care" as the name for our field. St. Christopher's was a hospice, and initially "hospice" was to be the name of the new program. However, Bal was cautioned by francophone colleagues that "hospice" had a negative connotation in the French language, conveying a disengagement from life.

He tells me he was pondering this conundrum in the shower one day and the phrase "palliative care" popped into his fertile mind—and thus "palliative care" entered our lexicon. This term was initially opposed by Dame Cicely and British colleagues, but ultimately accepted. It began to be used internationally, and to this day it is the flag behind which we march.

1980s

In the early eighties I was working as director of the Cross Cancer Institute at the University of Alberta while also serving as secretary treasurer on the board of the American Society of Clinical Oncology (ASCO). I continued to think about Dr. Mount's palliative care program and decided I would return to Montreal to learn more. This news was met by some of my ASCO colleagues with puzzlement, by others with scorn and, in one case, outright anger. Many of my oncology colleagues saw no need for palliative care.

I started my new educational journey at St. Christopher's, where I first met Declan Walsh, and then studied and worked with Robert Twycross and Geoff Hanks at Oxford. I was privileged to next study with Kathy Foley at Memorial Sloan Kettering Cancer Center before returning to join Dr. Mount at McGill. I learned quite a lot from a most impressive faculty! Some years later, these relationships led me to become a coeditor of the *Oxford Textbook of Palliative Medicine* with Geoff Hanks and Derek Doyle.

Upon my return to Alberta, I started a palliative care program within my cancer center, which was not met with universal approval. When I coupled that decision with the inauguration of a division of psychology, I thought the radiologists and radiotherapists would draw and quarter me. Not a surprising view at that time. It was still the era of "kill-the-tumor," and oncologists were buoyed by our success in curing advanced testicular cancer as well as a range of hematologic and children's cancers. Many oncologists, overly optimistic about the rate of progress in curing advanced solid tumors, strongly opposed directing funds toward spiritual/psychosocial enterprises.

But a critical change in oncologists' attitudes had begun due to the breakdown of tribal thinking. Initially, we oncologists viewed ourselves as belonging to a separate tribe, with all the problems that come about when we regard people in other fields as alien, not sharing the wisdom of our tribe. Within cancer centers, communication with members of other oncology subspecialties was commonly substandard, resulting in patterns of care that today we regard as uniformly unacceptable. First the patient was seen by a surgeon or sometimes a radiotherapist, and then, if the disease was progressing, by medical-radiotherapy oncologists. And then, when our patients were dying, we muddled along as best we could. We oncologists did finally come to learn that early joint consultation by a surgeon, radiotherapist, and medical oncologist working as a team was essential; witness the success of adjuvant therapy at the onset of treatment. Notably, these teams still did not include colleagues from the newly developing field of palliative care. Oncologists thought that palliative care was soft, not directly addressing the cancer and thus not worthy of an invitation into the care of patient and family until the very end of life.

One reason they dismissed palliative care is that unlike traditional oncology, it did not have a firm research infrastructure. Progress in a medical discipline is dependent on a sound research foundation. Palliative care's foundation was very modest. There was a wealth of wisdom and informed opinion but little in the way of evidence-based practice.

Palliative care research faced many hurdles. Most of us had little training in methodology, and we worried about ethical issues related to informed consent and causing patient-family distress. We wished to protect our patients, not recognizing that ethical research could be done and that our patients would welcome participation, seeing themselves as advancing common human well-being. Granting agencies followed traditional patterns of funding; they were only interested in research attacking cancer tissue and regarded symptom research as a subservient issue. The governing pattern of research was not patient-family based—they were not partners; rather, patients were passive recipients of therapies, which they did not often understand well.

A turning point for me, which ultimately also contributed to the growing respect for our field, came in 1984 with the recruitment of Eduardo Bruera to a fellowship post at the Cross Cancer Institute at the University of Alberta. One day I received Eduardo's CV from the head of the Canadian National Cancer Institute. This young Argentinian was only in his twenties; he had already published seminal articles on the use of corticosteroids in symptom management and on autonomic system dysfunction. I encouraged him to join us in Edmonton as a fellow, and within a few months the "fellow" was establishing a flourishing palliative care research program with studies on opioids, hydration, and autonomic effects on gastric emptying, among others, and teaching me clinical research. At that time Dr. Foley and colleagues such as Dr. Russ Portenoy were conducting a series of seminal studies giving us the expertise to control cancer pain. Jimmie Holland forged the field of psycho-oncology, introducing us to research on psychosocial issues that buttressed the fundamental tenets of palliative care. These leaders, together with Dr. Mount, taught and inspired others to enrich our research initiatives then and indeed to this day.

In the 1980s, the World Health Organization (WHO) became an early convert in support of palliative care. Under the leadership of a charismatic, visionary Swede, Jan Stjernswärd, a radiotherapist by training, the WHO cancer division changed its name to the Cancer and Palliative Care Division. Before joining the WHO, Jan had worked in Kenya, where he was sensitized to the suffering of patients dying in pain without access to opioids or any other drug that might lessen pain. Clearly for everyone, but particularly for people suffering in underdeveloped nations, palliative care had to be a major part of a cancer program. In 1989, I was on a WHO task force, chaired by Kathy Foley, which published a monograph, *Cancer Pain Relief and Palliative Care*. In this monograph we described palliative care as "the active total care of patients whose disease is not responsive to curative treatment. Control of pain, of other symptoms, and of psychological, social and spiritual problems is paramount.... Many aspects of palliative care are also applicable earlier in the course of the illness, in conjunction with anticancer treatment."[1] In these early times the report endorsed the early application of palliative care, a concept that finally found legs more than two decades later.

Among others, Kathy, with the later support of the Soros Open Society, alongside Jan, took on the mission of introducing palliative care to health systems throughout the world. Liliana DeLima, the executive director of the International Association for Hospice and Palliative Care, can attest to the success of these endeavors.

1990s

In sharp contrast to my 1980 ASCO experience, ASCO over the next two decades made a *volte-face*, ultimately becoming a champion for palliative care in all its dimensions (physical, social, emotional, and spiritual), as evidenced by the eventual inclusion of a palliative care and symptom control

section in the annual ASCO meeting, and welcoming palliative care specialists as speakers. ASCO introduced the patient-friendly CancerNet website,
and in a 1998 position paper on care at the end of life gave support for a close
liaison between oncologists and palliative care colleagues.[2] In 2009 the American Society of Clinical Oncology officially stated that palliative and spiritual
care are integral parts of cancer care and that the principles of palliative care
should be applied when a diagnosis of life-threatening illness is first made.[3]
This was further affirmed by ASCO in 2017. Indeed, today European[4] and
Australasian societies are aligned with ASCO, and some countries in the
middle-income and developing world have followed the WHO in including comprehensive palliative care in their nation's health policy mandate. In
2018, the Canadian Parliament passed a bill entitled *An Act Providing for the
Development of a Framework for Palliative Care in Canada.*

A NEW CENTURY

In the last ten years of my oncology odyssey, I have noted a further breakdown
of tribal walls. There is consensus that palliative care is not just an end-of-life
field; rather, early palliative care should be applied at the first diagnosis of a
predictably fatal illness. Since everyone is now on board, why has rhetoric not
matched reality? We still seem to have a long way to go to complete acceptance and integration of palliative care into oncology practice.

I think that four factors are slowing progress and prolonging the journey
to full integration. The first is the challenge of changing the massive inertia
of organizational cultures; the big dog still eats first. The needed change in
health care organization is a complex topic unto itself, which I will not attempt
to cover today.

A second factor is the primacy of the pharmaceutical industry in cancer
research and care. There is a strong pharmaceutical medical industrial complex. An article published in *Annals of Oncology* noted that two-thirds of
recent cancer research studies published in our leading journals, *Lancet* and
the *NEJM*, were funded by drug firms.[5] The prime objective of that research is
marketing new successful drugs. God bless them—they want to improve life,
both quality and quantity—but they also must increase shareholder wealth.
It is difficult to introduce palliative care research concepts into their studies,

and they still dominate clinical research. How to change that story is, as with the first factor, a big issue unto itself.

A third factor, notwithstanding ASCO's views, is the unchanging attitude of some oncologists linked to practice realities. Some practicing oncologists feel they are driving the bus and do not need and may not be able to sustain the seeming complexity of early palliative care integration.[6]

The fourth and final factor for lack of full integration of palliative care with oncology is the slow appreciation of newer research about cancer biology. Too many oncologists compartmentalize cancer progression and symptom progression in two different buckets. However, it is increasingly clear that the same etiologies drive both cancer symptoms and cancer growth. We have known for years that anti-inflammatory measures such as exercise, diet, and psychosocial well-being lower the risk of getting cancer, and more recently we have found that they are key in designing supportive care programs for patients treated with cure in mind, after completion of their primary therapy. It is not surprising that the same factors would play a role in patients with advanced cancer.

THE FUTURE

No longer should we regard addressing psychosocial issues and spiritual needs as simply comforting the patient and family while the "real stuff"—chemo/immunotherapy—proceeds apace. Today we know that brain processes, stress, and an immune system turned traitorous are major drivers of cancer growth, but the same processes are in a major way responsible for causing patient physical and psychosocial symptoms and suffering. Palliative care therapies, including social and spiritual support, nutrition, exercise, other anti-inflammatory measures, and excellent symptom control, can reduce stress and return abnormal immune-endocrine stimuli toward normal.

Some of that work comes from Susan Lutgendorf and her colleagues, who have shown the deleterious effects of human stress. In a *JCO* article, they state that "in vitro, in vivo, and clinical studies show that stress related processes can impact pathways implicated in cancer progression including immune regulation, angiogenesis, and invasion."[7] A subsequent "Snapshot" publication summarizes the varied pathophysiologic aberrations induced by stress and point out that these effects can also influence the incidence and progression of other chronic, ultimately fatal diseases.[8] It is not a platitude that the advanced cancer patient and family should be embraced in a care plan with spiritual, psychosocial, and blended oncology palliative components and care; it makes sound scientific sense.

This new concept requires a multimodal team model of care and research. While the team may vary in membership, a multimodal team departs from the traditional nurse/physician dyad and will include social workers, psychologists, spiritual care personnel, and the patient and family as full participants. I would also add nutritionists and physio-occupational therapists. I have noted how this invitation to be part of the team is clearly welcomed by patients, and perhaps more so by families.[9] Here, they truly are active team members, as key therapies such as nutrition, exercise, and spiritual care enlist their participation. That early palliative care improves quality of life is now a given, but might early palliative care also increase *quantity* of life? I believe so. It is proven in animal models (yes, tranquil care can improve survival)[10] and demonstrated in at least a few human studies. What we know about the new cancer biology should demand that we move from rhetoric to open the door to fully integrated care and research systems.

I had the good fortune to sit down with Dr. Mount for a three-hour chat a few months before starting this essay. We talked of many things— what a remarkable opportunity to spend time with this remarkable man. We went over our experience, and I asked him what he thought of our future. Bal brought me back to the beginning of his work at St. Christopher's and stated that as it was then so it must continue. It is key that we not lose the spiritual-existential dimension of palliative care.

Some years ago, Bal penned a thoughtful personal narrative, "The Existential Moment." In it he states, "in accompanying those who are dying over the past quarter century I have come to view life as a spiritual experience, that is to say, a search for meaning, purpose, and personal connection to something greater and more enduring than the self."[11] In our recent conversation he expanded on this theme, stating, "Our success in assisting our patients and their families (not to mention ourselves) hasn't changed in the decades since St Christopher's opened in 1967, the key determinant in influencing quality and I daresay quantity of life remains our full understanding of the interdependence of the four domains that interact to define human experience—Physical, Psychological, Social and Existential/Spiritual. To ignore one of these aspects of our consciousness is to unintentionally hamstring our outcome."[12]

NOTES

1. World Health Organization 1990, 11.
2. American Society of Clinical Oncology 1998.
3. Ferris et al. 2009.
4. Jordan et al. 2018.
5. Dogan, Yamamoto-Ibusuki, and Andre 2018.
6. Kruser et al. 2018.
7. Lutgendorf, Sood, and Antoni 2010.
8. Archana et al. 2016.
9. Chasen, Bhargava, and MacDonald 2014.
10. Riley 1975.
11. Mount 2003, 94.
12. I commend to anyone wanting to read even more deeply on this subject Dr. Balfour Mount's recently published memoir, *Ten Thousand Crossroads: The Path as I Remember It* (Montreal: McGill-Queen's University Press, 2020), which contains the clearest exposition of the importance of spirituality in medical care that I have ever read.

WORKS CITED

American Society of Clinical Oncology. 1998. "Cancer Care During the Last Phase of Life." *Journal of Clinical Oncology* 16 (5): 1986–96.

Archana, S. N., N. C. Sadaoui, P. L. Dorniak, S. K. Lutgendorf, and A. K. Sood. 2016. "Snapshot: Stress and Disease." *Cell Metabolism* 23 (2): 388.

Chasen, M., R. Bhargava, and N. MacDonald. 2014. "Rehabilitation for Patients with Advanced Cancer." *CMAJ* 186 (14): 1071–75.

Dogan, S., M. Yamamoto-Ibusuki, and F. Andre. 2018. "Funding Sources of Practice-Changing Trials." *Annals of Oncology* 29 (4): 1063–65.

Ferris, F. D., E. Bruera, N. Cherny, C. Cummings, D. Currow, D. Dudgeon, N. Janjan, F. Strasser, C. F. von Gunten, and J. H. Von Roenn. 2009. "Palliative Cancer Care a Decade Later: Accomplishments, the Need, Next Steps—from the American Society of Clinical Oncology." *Journal of Clinical Oncology* 27 (18): 3052–58.

Jordan, K., M. Aapro, S. Kaasa, C. I. Ripamonti, F. Scotté, F. Strasser, A. Young, E. Bruera, J. Herrstedt, D. Keefe, B. Larid, D. Walsh, J. Y. Douillard, and A. Cervantes. 2018. "European Society for Medical Oncology (ESMO) Position Paper on Supportive and Palliative Care." *Annals of Oncology* 29 (1): 36–43.

Kruser, T. J., J. M. Kruser, J. Gross, M. Moran, K. Kaiser, E. Szmuilowicz, and S. Mehta Kircher. 2018. "Barriers to Early Integration of Palliative Care: A Qualitative Analysis of Medical Oncologist Attitudes and Practice Patterns." *Journal of Clinical Oncology* 36 (15 suppl.).

Lutgendorf, S. K., A. K. Sood, and M. H. Antoni. 2010. "Host Factors and Cancer Progression: Biobehavioral Signaling Pathways and Interventions." *Journal of Clinical Oncology* 28 (26): 4094–99.

Mount, B. M. 2003. "The Existential Moment." *Palliative and Supportive Care* 1 (1): 93–96.

Riley, V. 1975. "Mouse Mammary Tumors: Alteration of Incidence as Apparent Function of Stress." *Science* 189 (4201): 465–67.

World Health Organization. 1990. *Cancer Pain Relief and Palliative Care.* World Health Organization Technical Report Series 804. Geneva: World Health Organization.

CHAPTER 4

Palliative Medicine

A Personal Journey

Declan Walsh

SO FAR, SO GOOD?

One of my first medical school clinical experiences was a visit to Our Lady's Hospice in Harold's Cross, Dublin. Religious statuary, a somewhat morbid atmosphere, and a distinct cultural difference from the general hospital ward remain imprinted in my memory to this day, fifty years after graduating from University College Dublin Medical School in 1971. I completed an internship at St. Vincent's University Hospital but found the educational, social, and intellectual atmosphere of the time there stifling. Searching for a different experience, I came to the States for two years before moving to the United Kingdom to pursue a master's degree in clinical biochemistry with a pharmacology focus.[1]

During those years, I gained insight into what was less interesting to me—dermatology, hypertension research—and what was more interesting—internal medicine and geriatrics. I also developed an interest in business management theory, à la Peter Drucker, as well as military history and rock music. I still ponder the link between those three disparate interests.

THE GEORDIES

Following completion of my master's work, I entered a two-year internal medicine and geriatrics rotation as a senior house officer in Newcastle-on-Tyne.

Then as now, academics interested me, so I published my first bit of academic writing, a letter[2] to the *New England Journal of Medicine*—quite exciting so early in one's career! During that time, I happened upon my second exposure to hospice, this time a lunchtime educational movie on the subject (St. Christopher's Hospice). The idea resonated but did not yet stick with me. I began to plan for a return to the United States (or perhaps Ireland) to pursue general hospital medicine.

SERENDIPITY AND A MOVIE

One day, I chanced to look at the *British Medical Journal* jobs listing and saw a posting for a clinical pharmacology research fellow (on analgesics for cancer pain) at the same St. Christopher's Hospice (SCH) in London. I remembered Our Lady's Hospice in Dublin and the movie in Newcastle-on-Tyne. As it happened, I had a free afternoon and went to visit the hospice, an intimate setting compared to the hospitals I had worked in, which was somewhat oddly located on a typical suburban road in southeast London. There I first met Cicely Saunders and was immediately impressed by her vision, energy, and humor. Investigating opiates and antidepressants seemed much more exotic than the typical clinical pharmacology job of addressing high blood pressure. So I decided to apply and was successful. There were two candidates; the other went on to a distinguished career in palliative medicine in the UK.

ANOTHER WORLD

I have often said that I went to St. Christopher's for an afternoon but stayed four years. Saunders had a clear vision that to develop hospice it needed an evidence base.[3] She herself had done some elementary clinical research and was prepared to commit resources—no doubt scarce—to a research fellow. A prior fellow (Robert Twycross) had successfully completed an MD thesis on the use of morphine and heroin for cancer pain. After he left, there was a hiatus. Robert had done excellent work, but the research activities were wound down after his departure. A successor had tragically committed suicide (in the hospice), and I was, as I learned later, his replacement!

HOW TO DO IT AND HOW NOT TO DO IT

The task therefore was not only to set up the actual projects but also to reconstitute a small research unit, which unfortunately took considerable time and energy away from the research itself. The appointment was in collaboration with the London Hospital Clinical Pharmacology Unit, which had an interest in clinical trials and biostatistics. The ethical, practical, and logistical difficulties of conducting research in the hospice soon became apparent.[4] There was no one on hospice staff who had any significant research experience. Various advisers were both smart and well-intended, but (I thought) impractical about the realities of the patient population.

The senior hospice clinical physicians at that time were Dr. Mary Baines and Dr. Tom West.[5] They exemplified the best of English medical practice. I learned much from their clinical wisdom and the ideas they championed: careful clinical observation of the patient, astute physical examination skills, common sense, and *a willingness to challenge medical orthodoxy*.[6] Some of the hospice staff were less enamored of the proposed research. I found this frustrating. There was a sense of what we now call gatekeeping; research might be admirable in theory but not in reality!

Establishing the research unit was an uphill battle,[7] but the task was significantly assisted by my prior interest in management theory. To my surprise, I discovered that I had a talent for concise medical scientific writing and protocol design. We obtained a grant from the (then) Department of Health and Social Security. It soon became evident, however, that the research was overly ambitious. There was neither the research culture nor organizational sophistication to successfully execute the planned projects—particularly with a novice research fellow! Indeed, the issues we grappled with have continued to challenge the entire field of palliative medicine research until now, including clinical trial design, patient accrual, dropout rates, and generalizability of results. No doubt I did not make matters any easier, as I had a short fuse and was impatient to get things done and go back to the United States.

MENTORS AND LEADERS

The work was complex due to a combination of my inexperience in clinical research, the major challenges inherent in the proposed work, and the well-meaning naïveté of some of my advisors. I was also now professionally isolated from the hurly-burly of the teaching hospital environment, not part of a larger research unit—where I would have learned lessons from peers and avoided mistakes. As I progressed with two (overly ambitious) randomized controlled studies, one on tricyclic antidepressants, the other on sustained-release morphine, I became increasingly interested in the now evident wider complexities of cancer care.[8]

My time at SCH also exposed me to many other ideas and professionals with similar or related interests. Colin Murray-Parkes was conducting groundbreaking research at St. Christopher's on bereavement, while at the same time others were pursuing insights into nerve damage in head and neck cancer via autopsy studies. This illustrated the breadth of vision that Saunders had and her willingness to explore what is even now largely uncharted territory.

On the personal front, I also was fortunate to meet many future leaders in the field both within the UK and internationally. Balfour Mount, as dynamic a figure in the field as I have ever come across, was certainly one. We attempted some collaborative projects together, and I subsequently investigated a job at his unit in Montreal. Although unable to pursue that opportunity, I learned much from seeing his "palliative care unit" within a general hospital, and ten years later it became the basis for the acute care palliative medicine unit in Cleveland that we created in 1994.

Most significantly, while at SCH, I learned directly from Cicely Saunders. The evident attention to detail in every aspect of St. Christopher's was striking. This included interdisciplinary team meetings, management meetings (sometimes fueled by moderate amounts of alcohol), emphasis on first-rate nursing care, inclusion of art and music, architectural design, kind and visible leadership, and a thoughtful, incremental approach to program development. The difficulties she overcame to develop SCH must have been enormous.

She had various aphorisms that I have carried with me, such as "If you can't do everything, that doesn't mean you can't do something." I believe her brother (whom I never met) was a management consultant, and she frequently referred to his advice. We met regularly; these conversations stood me in good stead in my later management years at the Cleveland Clinic[9] and added to the management insights learned from Peter Drucker.

OUT OF THE FRYING PAN, INTO THE FIRE

During my time at SCH, I realized the complexity of advanced cancer both from a psychological and physical viewpoint.[10] I was also sensitized by the hospice culture to the wider challenges for the patient and family. I resolved that I would make this my career. At the time, there was no "palliative medicine" subspecialty and thus no fellowship. The only apparent option was to train in medical oncology. To do this in the UK was challenging; priority was given to local graduates and required a lengthy commitment. Medical oncology fellowships in the United States, in contrast, were no longer than three years, so I applied to multiple cancer centers in the United States and Canada. At that time, it was possible to buy a "round-robin" ticket to visit multiple cities, which is what I did: Boston, Buffalo, Houston, New York, Rochester (Minnesota), Toronto, and Washington, DC. It was a whirlwind tour; I stayed in each city for one day. Some were clearly bemused by my interest in treating the patient rather than the cancer. I was fortunate to be offered several positions, and it came down to a choice between Mayo Clinic and Memorial Sloan Kettering Cancer Center. The latter had the attraction of New York and the bonus of the famed cancer pain service, which involved Kathleen Foley, Ray Houde, Chuck Inturrisi, Bob Kaiko, and Ada Rogers. I had had some contact with these folks during my tenure at SCH; it looked like a win-win. The proposed fellowship was in medical oncology with a specific interest in clinical pharmacology, so it appeared the stars were aligned. We decided on New York City.

Despite all that I was learning at SCH, I decided to switch gears and obtained an additional honorary appointment at Guy's Hospital in the unit led by Professor John Trounce. He had edited a classic book on medicine (that I had used as an undergraduate) and was widely admired and regarded as "a wise bird." We did some pharmacokinetic work on morphine and its metabolites, some of which was ultimately published in abstract and letter form.[11] I had learned a lot and admired the English (and Scottish) approach to medicine, but I did not see a long-term future in the UK. Having said that, I left for the United States before it was wise to do so; this was a significant career error, since much of my work done at SCH was never formally published.[12] I should have stayed another six months and completed it. Instead, impatient, I set off with a young family to New York City.

A TOUGH TOWN

We spent Christmas 1979 in Dublin and, on December 26, flew to New York. The intent was to start work on January 1. On arrival in the city (with a one-year-old), we discovered that my department had forgotten to arrange an apartment across the road from the hospital that was typically provided for fellows. We obtained private accommodation after significant hassle and later moved into a hospital apartment. The weather was a shock, too, as it was the coldest winter in New York for a century. My orientation to Memorial Hospital was by the chief fellow, who took me to a room, kicked the door of one of the lockers, said, "This is yours," and promptly left.

I was assigned to the Section of Developmental Chemotherapy as a special fellow but would participate in all the usual medical oncology fellowship training. This consisted of eighteen months of clinical rotations in medical oncology (but not hematology, which I disliked). Despite the somewhat rocky start, I quickly settled in and thoroughly enjoyed the interactions, the training, and the rapid learning curve. Although some unspecified interaction with the cancer pain service led by Kathleen Foley had been discussed during my interviews, it was (disappointingly) made very clear shortly after I started that I was to focus exclusively upon developmental chemotherapy—and stay away from the pain service.

The culture and day-to-day operations of the hospital in New York were a total change from SCH. While clinical care was excellent, the motto was "Push that chemo." Concepts of palliative care at that time were simply not part of the conversation. Patients came from far and wide to get cured. They were prepared to endure significant discomfort, expense, and morbidity in pursuit of that goal. This reinforced the attitudes of clinical staff, no matter how unrealistic cure might be. The sense was that everyone was involved in an enterprise whose ultimate goal was to cure cancer. Any other considerations were distinctly secondary. "Shake and bake" described patients' adverse reactions to antifungal medications often prescribed as a consequence of chemotherapy-induced neutropenic sepsis. In addition, this was also a time when many inpatients were suffering from the infectious and carcinogenic complications of the early AIDS epidemic. Unusual infections, complications, and tumors were the order of the day.

BIG PHARMA AND MEDICAL PUBLISHING

I was involved in the conduct of both clinical and pharmacokinetic studies of Phase I chemotherapy agents.[13] This took place largely after the first eighteen months of the fellowship. I learned liquid chromatography to measure drug levels of two agents: merbarone and trimethrexate. The discipline and structure of Phase I clinical studies were interesting. Significant patient toxicities were part of, and essential to, the investigative process. There was also the opportunity to work with people, most of whom were world famous in their fields. It was just an extraordinary experience. Simply put, I loved Memorial Sloan Kettering and New York City.

During the latter part of my fellowship, I came into contact with some of the companies who manufactured analgesics. One of their affiliates in the UK had provided limited research support for a study I conducted there. I was contacted by another U.S.-based company, which was developing a sustained-release morphine formulation. I designed some of their studies (based on my original protocol from London) and acted as a consultant and site coordinator for studies in Detroit, Denver, Lexington, and various other locations. At the same time, I was involved in analyzing and publishing the Phase I data from the Sloan Kettering Memorial studies. I also had approached publishers in London about a potential book. This (*Symptom Control*, published by Blackwell in 1989) came to fruition during my time in New York; I edited and contributed to that book during my fellowship.[14] (My wife Cora and a friend helped type the manuscript.) With my ever-growing interest in pain management in cancer patients, I began work with others on new ideas like subcutaneous opioid infusions via patient-controlled analgesia.[15]

PALLIATIVE MEDICINE EMERGES

During my time at Memorial Sloan Kettering, I met many others who would lead the development of hospice and, later, palliative medicine in the United States and elsewhere. I reconnected with Balfour Mount and for the first time met Neil MacDonald, whose unit in Edmonton I visited. I participated with Josefina Magno in some of the early meetings of what later became the American Academy of Hospice and Palliative Medicine. During that time, initiatives in the UK and other European countries led to the development of the field of palliative medicine. Geoff Hanks, with whom I had overlapped during my tenure in St. Christopher's, was very important in this regard. He had been a research fellow with Robert Twycross in Oxford after Robert left SCH. At the time, I was unaware of these developments, as I had lost contact with SCH, erstwhile colleagues, and others in Europe. I was totally consumed by the personal and professional challenges of our new life in the United States.

SLIDING DOOR: THE MOVIE IN REAL LIFE

As my fellowship at Memorial Sloan Kettering drew to a close, the question arose as to what to do next, so I investigated opportunities in Canada and the United States. I was also offered a position in Memorial Sloan Kettering as a junior attending and, on a particular day in late 1986, was to sign a contract with John Mendelsohn, who was then chief physician—before he moved to MD Anderson in Houston. That morning, I was on rounds and realized I had left a draft manuscript in my apartment across the street. I ran across, but no one was home, and, as I hurried out the door, the telephone rang. It was the Cleveland Clinic inquiring about a leadership position to develop a "palliative care service." It was exactly the opportunity I was seeking. I subsequently interviewed in Cleveland, was offered the position, and accepted with a start date of August 1, 1987.

I had deferred on a decision about New York until things were clarified in Cleveland; everyone at Memorial was gracious about this. One of the attending physicians, however, laughed out loud when I told him I was moving from Manhattan to Cleveland. This was a little disconcerting. I had little knowledge of Cleveland or its somewhat negative reputation because of economic decline, particularly since the race riots of the 1960s. While the Memorial position was exciting, it was not exactly what I wanted to do. I decided to pursue my passion at the Cleveland Clinic, which seemed to offer the best combination of personal circumstances and professional opportunities. It later emerged that John Raaf, chairman of the Cleveland Clinic Cancer Center, had contacted Kathleen Foley, who recommended me for consideration.

SERENDIPITY STRIKES AGAIN: THE CLEVELAND CLINIC (1987–1994)

John Raaf had worked at Memorial—hence the contact with Kathleen Foley. The department included both oncology and hematology and (at the time) was small. I was assigned to the outpatient clinic, where I did general medical oncology with an emphasis on lung cancer based on my Memorial work. It was understood that I would develop a palliative care service. I had little understanding of what such a service might look like, nor did anyone at the Clinic articulate what it would involve! A needs assessment (later published) had been done prior to my arrival. This had been stimulated by an unfortunate sequence of events with a particular patient where clinical care in pain control had been badly handled.

Fortunately, I had negotiated as part of my recruitment that two RNs would be provided to help structure the new service. These were duly appointed, and we announced the creation of a palliative care inpatient consult service and started seeing patients in the late summer and early fall of 1987. Two things were done at the start that had a major impact later: first, we started collecting detailed information about the number and types of patients referred, and second, we developed a business plan.[16] These stood us in good stead as the program grew in volume and complexity.[17]

The Cleveland Clinic has been associated over many years with innovation in medicine. The administrative structure includes physician leadership as a key concept at all levels (including the CEO). In addition, physician executive leaders are appointed based firstly upon acknowledged clinical excellence, and most—even at senior levels—continued some clinical practice despite significant administrative responsibilities. This made the development of a new service much easier. I have no doubt that, at the time, it would have been impossible in any comparable organization with nonclinical leadership, due to their lack of clinical insight and experience.

PROGRAM DEVELOPMENT

We started getting regular consultations (particularly for pain control) and continued our efforts to market the service with leaflets, personal contacts, and presentations to interested groups.[18] It was clear that there were many clinicians who were enthusiastic but also some who were quite hostile. During that time and in subsequent years, there were a (very) few physician colleagues who did much to try and inhibit the growth of the program and damage its development in many small ways. In retrospect, I believe they believed that the hostility would wear me down and I would quit. This was disheartening and very stressful. I quickly learned to focus on the positive rather than spin my wheels with those who did not have our best interests at heart.

We began getting requests to follow patients after hospital discharge and so decided to open dedicated outpatient clinics integrated into the usual Cancer Center medical oncology clinics, but which specialized in palliative medicine. These hours, on Tuesday and Thursday afternoons, became extremely busy. In turn, they started to attract outpatient consultations from within the Cancer Center and not just follow-up hospital discharges. As we became busier, I was still scheduled as a medical oncologist in the outpatient setting; this responsibility started to interfere with our inpatient service. After some tension with the medical oncology department chair, it was agreed to free me up to spend more time on palliative medicine; this arrangement continued for several years on an approximately fifty-fifty basis. As a result, the inpatient consult service grew rapidly in 1988 and 1989.

TAKEOFF

It quickly became clear that referring services were increasingly relying on our advice and orders in routine inpatient management.[19] We were in effect managing care even though not the physician of record. This had multiple implications in workload on individual patients, as we were effectively responsible for most aspects of their day-to-day clinical care. In addition, we were now looking after patients all over the hospital, so considerable time was spent on rounds. Furthermore, concerns arose when we were not available and visible on the weekends, so I started rounding on Saturday and Sunday mornings.

Unfortunately, this became an exhausting commitment, which continued for over five years and at some level from which I never really personally recovered. This situation improved later, with the addition of an (unaccredited) clinical fellowship position[20] in palliative medicine, which allowed me to round just six days a week! Clinical volumes continued to grow, so the addition of one fellow was only a relative advantage. Simultaneously we received requests to assume primary care responsibility for many of the consultations.

This was a double-edged sword: on one level, it was often less work to take care of the issues ourselves, but it was also more responsibility to be the primary service. In addition, for several years, I was on call every night (including weekends). By now I was bored with the chemotherapy side of things and elected to discontinue my lung cancer practice and focus on "palliative care."

Although I was unaware of it then, the business model of the Cleveland Clinic was under stress because of changed reimbursement, coupled with increased demands of the federal bureaucracy, such as increased regulatory intrusion and supervision. This resulted in a change of leadership and the appointment of a new CEO, Dr. Fred Loop, a cardiac surgeon. He made wide-ranging changes to medical operations, the community footprint, philanthropy, education, and research. He was aggressive and could be abrasive. To me, he seemed to be a natural CEO, although he had had no formal business training. The chief of staff was Dr. Ralph Straffon, a urological surgeon. I made it my business to make the new leadership aware of the various program developments. This attracted some further scrutiny, mostly welcome, some unwelcome! In a conversation with Ralph (later a president of the American College of Surgeons), it emerged that he had a daughter who had died from leukemia. Because that had been a terrible experience, he encouraged me to pursue my plans vigorously and said that that he would "look out for me"—or words to that effect (which he did)—in the event of any political opposition or naysaying by colleagues.

LIFE-WORK LESSONS

When I was a fellow at Memorial Sloan Kettering, we had already had three children, one of whom, at the age of two and a half, started to exhibit behavioral changes of concern. We did not know it at the time, but he was one of those children who typified the huge apparent increase in the incidence of autism; he was on the leading wave of that development. This was a life-changing event for our entire family, although this did not become fully apparent until some years later, when the severity and extent of his disability was fully recognized.

Largely due to the heroic actions of my wife, he is now a contented and involved adult living on a farm in western Ohio specifically designed for adults with autism. We had over two decades of challenging times with our son because of his disruptive and sometimes bizarre autism behaviors, which had inevitably severe and far-reaching deleterious effects on our family life and two other sons. I also, however, learned an enormous amount from the experience and hope that it made me a better person (and a better physician). Specifically, it brought home in a very real way the importance of the dignity of the individual and the realization that every life has value; the integrity of each life must be respected and enhanced, no matter how difficult the circumstances. It further sensitized me to the important dynamics between physical and psychological illnesses and socioeconomic status.

It had become clear that our son was severely autistic and disabled in terms of behavior, cognitive function, social interaction, and speech. My wife worked tirelessly to deal with the situation, as little was known about autism at the time. Nevertheless, she accessed resources such as music therapy, which not only benefited my son but also widened my perspectives around the great value such services could provide.[21] I subsequently applied these lessons to the palliative care service, including the introduction of music therapy to the Cleveland Clinic as a formal structured program—where it has prospered. This was before the concept of work-life balance; suffice it to say that the challenges of that time and for many years subsequently regarding my professional life were significant. The cumulative stress, time pressures, lack of sleep, and long hours at work, with little real downtime at home, were enormously difficult, particularly with a new service and a new concept of cancer care—an uphill struggle even in the best of circumstances.

HOSPICE MEDICAL DIRECTOR

By 1992, we had a well-established inpatient consultation service, inpatient palliative medicine service, and outpatient clinics integrated within the Cancer Center day-to-day operations. We experienced difficulty accessing local hospice services and also discovered a somewhat adversarial approach concerning the care of patients whom we referred.[22] This was an unpleasant surprise, as we regarded ourselves not just as a source of referrals but also as a source of specific expertise in the area! This became an operational concern; in response I developed a business plan so that the Clinic could start its own hospice service. This was approved after the usual administrative and executive scrutiny and was developed in collaboration with existing Cleveland Clinic Home

Care services. This was important because it provided a guaranteed revenue stream credited to the palliative care service and was a demonstrable hospital benefit in more effective discharges and fewer readmissions. I believe we were the only major medical center in the United States that managed and owned our own hospice; usually these were community-based endeavors. Apart from the logistical and financial advantages, this arrangement created tremendous operational continuity of patient care between inpatient, outpatient, and home.

It had become my practice wherever possible to do occasional home visits for individual patients, particularly Cleveland Clinic staff members or others seriously ill at home. One day I got a call from Dr. Ralph Straffon about a patient named Harry Horvitz. Mr. Horvitz was a well-respected local businessman with advanced prostate cancer, bone metastases, and severe pain. Fortunately, we controlled his pain with a subcutaneous patient-controlled analgesia pump. He was a very engaging gentleman; he liked the way I dressed, and I admired his interest in Western movies. I visited him at home on several occasions and met his wife, Lois.

BUSINESS PLANS AND MONEY MATTERS

As we proceeded with program development, I reached back to my interest in Peter Drucker's books on management.[23] I resolved to demonstrate that there was both a business and a humanitarian case for palliative medicine. Accordingly, for each new service line we had a business plan to convince decision-makers.[24] This was effective; it demonstrated a seriousness and clarity of purpose. In addition, we had an overarching business plan developed in collaboration with colleagues in nursing, finance, and administration (and subsequently published in a medical journal). This allowed us to establish relationships with key decision-makers in the organization.[25] Some may have had significant reservations about what was proposed—but at least saw we were well organized!

In addition to the business plans, we implemented several organizational structures and operational innovations within the service.[26] These included daily team huddles, which reviewed the clinical events of the previous twenty-four hours; a weekly administrative meeting, which reviewed the prior seven days; a quarterly business plan review; and regular retreats to keep us on track. All of these were conducted using templated agendas and structured conduct and follow-up. Indirectly, these burnished our reputation, but they also meant that we (usually) were well prepared for any challenges that came our way.[27] I also paid a lot of attention to financial analysis, as it was evident that, while we were not expected to make a lot of money for the organization, there was no desire for us to lose money either! The repeated need to justify our existence from a financial perspective was very wearing, but we made a virtue of necessity.[28] I learned not to trust any financial data provided unless I vetted it myself. This reinforced my (still held) conviction that a clinical leader with an interest in administrative matters could be a powerful force.

PHILANTHROPY

We developed an advisory board of interested individuals who provided advice on program development, helped us organize fundraiser events, and donated money to support the program. The board was chaired by a local businessman named Jerry Burkons, who also sponsored a lecture series for invited national and international experts in palliative medicine to visit the clinic. Mr. Burkons later established an endowed chair for the program. One of the visitors, Jan Stjernswärd, was from the World Health Organization cancer unit; subsequently I visited him in Geneva, and we were awarded a World Health Organization designation as a Demonstration Project in Palliative Care. This was gratifying but more important politically, as the senior administration was delighted with the honor, which cemented our reputation as a good program.

BURNOUT

A lot had been accomplished, but we were now at a crossroads. It was still a solo practice with only one attending physician and a large clinical workload. In addition, I had (belatedly) realized that the work itself was inherently and continuously stressful, as all patients had multisystem disease with severe complex psychological and physical symptoms, structural complications of metastatic disease, and complex psychosocial concerns—a powerful mix.

Unlike most areas of medical practice, there were no stable patients. Everybody (and their family) was a clinical challenge in some respect. The palliative care service was also the final common pathway after a lengthy complex illness. We often had to deal with issues around perceived or actual prior bad experiences or clinical mismanagement. This greatly added to the sense of stress and burnout. But things were about to change.

LOIS HORVITZ AND FAMILY

Harry Horvitz died in 1992. Following his death, I attended the gathering at his home and remember being impressed by the family group. Some months later, out of the blue, I received a call from his son Michael, who told me that a family business meeting had been held in which a decision was made to donate $1 million to the palliative care service. The object of the donation was to establish a specialist inpatient unit for palliative care. I was stunned.

We obtained preliminary cost estimates of $2 million to renovate a suitable area of the hospital. I approached Dr. Loop, who quickly agreed to match the Horvitz donation. An advisory board was established, chaired by the businessman and philanthropist Art Modell, but if I had to pick one community leader most responsible for working with me and others at the Cleveland Clinic to develop the palliative care unit, it would be Lois Horvitz.

Mrs. Horvitz committed her own personal time to the project, including working with the architect and the Clinic's construction management team. I had been put on notice by one of the Clinic leaders that Lois was (affectionately) "a pistol." She had worked previously with a cardiologist in the introduction of cardiopulmonary resuscitation to the United States. From that experience, she had little patience with medical conservatism. We got on well, with lots of laughs (but few disagreements) during a complex process in which she had a major personal and financial investment.

She had a wealth of thoughtful and creative ideas and arranged for an interior designer to participate. We conducted site visits (by private jet) to the palliative care unit at the Royal Victoria Hospital in Montreal, Calvary Hospital in New York, and Hospice of San Diego in California. Mrs. Horvitz also sourced furniture and fittings intended to soften the institutional nature of such a unit. Special attention was paid to colors, lighting, and noise reduction, as everyone realized that patients admitted to this unit very often would have had multiple prior admissions and were (often literally) sick of being in the hospital.

THE HORVITZ CENTER (1994–2012)

The unit, when it opened, was a stunning environment,[29] and I remained involved with it for eighteen years[30] as the medical director and, later, the Harry R. Horvitz Chair in Palliative Medicine—the first such chair in the United States. The original unit design served both patients and their families (and the staff) well over the ensuing years despite a high volume of traffic and busy patient environment. Many visitors came from across the country and around the world. Not everyone within the Cancer Center was enthusiastic. One or two colleagues were openly hostile, and no doubt others were opposed less publicly. I recognized what a bold move Fred Loop made in matching the donation. I have no doubt he got heat from irate surgical colleagues who probably thought he had lost his mind!

We had negotiated with the internal medicine program for internal residents to rotate through the unit to provide 24/7 coverage and to start including palliative medicine concepts in their training. The week before the unit was scheduled to open, a Cancer Center "colleague," who had temporary administrative responsibility, abruptly and without notice or discussion withdrew the residents. By this time, we had recruited a second attending physician (on a temporary contract) but were now faced with staffing a twenty-three-bed acute care unit for the sickest people in the hospital seven days a week, twenty-four hours a day, with only two attending physicians, one fellow, and no medical residents. In addition, we still had to provide our consultation service across the hospital, run outpatient clinics, and provide backup and medical cover for our hospice home care service. The day after the Horvitz Center opened, every bed was full. Little did I know at that time that some twenty-five years of successful operation later, in an act of medical administrative vandalism, the unit would be closed by a new cancer institute administrative leadership. It had been the first unit of its kind anywhere, with a special architectural design (the nursing staff designed the patient rooms). It included multiple physical elements to address the clinical, educational, and research activities focused on the needs of patients (and families) with advanced cancer. To my distress, it was replaced by a regular medical oncology unit.

HOME CARE

Hospice of the Cleveland Clinic opened in 1991. There were several local competitors, including a large, well-established community hospice, some of which appeared to be threatened by us. Our focus was, however, on Cleveland Clinic patients rather than the wider community. Cleveland Clinic Home Care had been developed and expanded rapidly in prior years. Yet because of changes in Medicare regulations, the business model became untenable, and Home Care ran into difficulties. Fred Loop asked me to go down to the administrative offices one day because of my interest in hospice home care.

When I arrived, it was clear that the organization was in disarray. There were three components: a Medicare-certified home care agency, a home pharmacy infusion, and durable medical equipment. I took over as chief executive officer and merged hospice with home care. We ultimately got the business back on track, expanded the geographical service area, and restored financial stability. Similarly, I became involved with the affiliated skilled nursing unit, which had fifty-nine beds. These were challenging executive roles because of complex reimbursement models, regulatory change, a chronically ill patient population, and a lack of appreciation for post-acute care among some of the administrative leadership. At a fundraiser event, Dr. Robert Kay, the dynamic new chief of staff of the Cleveland Clinic, suggested that a post-acute division be established, so I took the idea forward, obtained approval from the Cleveland Clinic board of governors with Dr. Loop's blessing, and became a division chair in 1995. The new division was to include home care and a long-term acute care hospital. It was also intended to develop services and relationships with other post-acute providers in the wider geographical area.

A WIDER ROLE

I took on these new responsibilities for several reasons. First, it was now clear that, to ensure the success of palliative medicine, it was important that I be a decision-maker rather than a decision-taker. Second, it was an opportunity to develop services that were philosophically and practically aligned in many ways with the developing field of palliative medicine, such as the importance of community care. Lastly, I liked the career opportunities and the authority that went with the responsibilities! Nevertheless, I still had a busy palliative medicine practice, was involved in research and academic publications, and lectured regularly outside the Cleveland Clinic, as well as participating in educational activities with the new clinical fellowship program in palliative medicine we had established.

At that time, I discovered during a checkup that my PSA (prostate-specific antigen) was slightly elevated. A subsequent recheck revealed it had risen again, and I was diagnosed with early stage moderately aggressive prostate cancer. This coincided with an unpleasant sequence of events, which included (in short order) the death of my father, major dental surgery, near death in car accidents (twice), and a major exacerbation of my son's difficulties with violent psychotic behavior. Given his illness, I opted for a definitive approach to the prostate cancer: radical prostatectomy. The early postoperative course was marked by severe bleeding and required significant transfusion support, but, aside from some minor complications, I returned to work three weeks later (a major mistake) out of concern for my colleagues' workload. By this time, we had added three attending physicians and had established a rotation system whereby one physician would be on the inpatient unit, one the consult service, and another the outpatient clinics.

During the same period, Dr. Loop resigned as CEO of the Cleveland Clinic, and I was not entirely satisfied with the consequences (I was an unsuccessful candidate for the role). The persistent understaffing of many of our areas of activity was a constant preoccupation and a drain on energy and morale. The combination of these chronic frustrations, the clinical and academic workload, and the challenges at home meant I was exhausted. As a result, I resigned from the editorial boards of several journals and roles with professional organizations; I was able to pass some of these responsibilities on to clinic colleagues.

On the outside, I was a division chair in a rapidly growing health system under the leadership of a now new and innovative CEO, a director and professor of an internationally known palliative medicine program with a strong track record of innovation, and a member of the board of governors of one of the top hospitals in the United States.

On the inside, I was psychologically and physically burnt out, with elements of posttraumatic stress disorder! I was simultaneously a section chief and chair in palliative medicine, as well as a division chair for a business that operated over a ten-thousand-square-mile area with, at any one time, a fourteen-thousand-patient census. I had also been elected to the board of governors of the Cleveland Clinic in 2004. The responsibilities on the board were significant. This involved annual professional reviews (an important part of the Clinic culture), chairing search committees for departments and divisions, and handling recruitment interviews and dinners. I was riding two horses: responsibilities of palliative medicine and an administrative role in the board of governors. The natural evolution entailed by the different priorities of the new CEO engendered a further sense of disorientation.

ANOTHER BOOK

Coincidentally, I was approached by a major publisher to act as editor for a textbook on palliative medicine.[31] At first uninterested, because of a prior unsatisfactory experience with the publishing industry, nevertheless I agreed, based upon assurances that we would innovate with an online book, which (in addition to the printed version) would be continuously updated. The book took about two years—the product of work early on Saturday and Sunday mornings—and was published in 2008. It sold well initially, received some good reviews, and was translated into Spanish, but the promised online component and continuous update never materialized to what had been envisioned, to my chagrin.

A BATTLE LOST

I completed my term on the board of governors at the Cleveland Clinic at the age of sixty-two in 2009. In the meantime, a new Cancer Center director, Dr. Derek Raghavan, had arrived from the University of Southern California. He was supportive of our activities in what was now a Section of Palliative Medicine based in the Horvitz Center, but we still faced major challenges in recruitment to match our clinical workload while we continued to publish aggressively on diverse topics in palliative medicine from infection to communication to anorexia and weight loss.[32] By this point, we had added a first-rate fellowship training program, a healthy hospice service, and an annual palliative medicine conference that drew both national and international attendees.

The Cleveland Clinic had been reorganized into institutes, replacing the previous division/department structure. I proposed that we create a

Rehabilitation Institute similar to the internationally famed one in Chicago. I was already the Physical Medicine Rehabilitation Department chair, and a business plan was prepared for the Rehabilitation Institute. Yet all was not well in the organization. We had, for example, developed two first-rate hospice units, one on either side of the city, to enable seriously ill patients to be discharged promptly to more appropriate and less costly care settings. However, both were closed abruptly by the administration without any consultation. The decision was simply handed down to us. Further, while informal approval had been given for the Rehabilitation Institute, the concept was later abandoned after what seemed to be an interminable delay, and the components of the preexisting post-acute division were broken up and distributed among the other new Institutes. Palliative medicine and the Horvitz Center would stay, I was told, in the new Cancer Institute. While all this chaos was going on, I was offered a visiting fellowship at Oxford University in the UK and, after some debate, was given approval by the clinic administration to go for six (not the original eight proposed by Oxford) weeks. In retrospect, I think this may have saved my life, as I only realized how debilitated I was after being there for some time.

BACK TO THE FUTURE

Later, I was asked to serve on a search committee for a new chair in palliative medicine in Dublin. The proposed chair was to be a joint venture between Trinity College Dublin and University College Dublin, my old medical school. One of the members of the search committee said, half-jokingly, "Why don't you do it?" I made the mistake of mentioning this to my wife, who also hailed from Dublin. Inevitably, when I reached retirement age, I submitted my resignation to the Cleveland Clinic after twenty-five years of service and took up the post in Dublin. I had come home, though not exactly.

Upon returning to Dublin, the first culture shock we felt was the deep economic distress caused by the crash of 2008, which flooded Ireland at the time. The second culture shock was the approach to academic activity of some within the hospice, where the professorship was physically based, even though I also had an office on the Trinity College campus. The administrator for the Research and Education facility within the hospice, where the new chair was to be located, met with me shortly after my arrival. She went to great pains to let me know all the things that she could not, and would not, do to assist me. This established the basis for our relationship for the ensuing four years; she was unwavering in her devotion to a fastidious lack of cooperation.

Even though the economy was on the ropes, it was clear that the chair represented a major opportunity because of the local talent available and the enormous resources in the two universities. I constructed a strategy, which initially focused on information technology applied to palliative medicine, particularly as pertaining to home care. There were two lecturer or senior registrar posts assigned to the chair, one from each of the universities. In addition to the information technology (IT) area, I elected to focus on the cancer weight-loss symptom complex (cachexia) and fatigue as major but poorly understood cancer symptom complexes.[33]

Funding was always a challenge. Atlantic Philanthropies was a major charity established by Chuck Feeney, who had decided to give away all his fortune before death. We submitted a successful grant application to Atlantic and were fortunate to receive a $1 million donation. This allowed us to expand the number of research fellow positions, and we embarked on an expanded research program in collaboration with various departments within both Trinity College Dublin and University College Dublin. This program is still in effect and due to be completed in 2024. Despite the administrative roadblocks, we also reorganized the undergraduate medical education for both medical schools in palliative medicine and developed a nationally webcast weekly palliative medicine grand rounds.

SUPPORTIVE ONCOLOGY

Meanwhile, I had trailing projects from the Cleveland Clinic that needed attention. Therefore, because of family commitments, I regularly traveled between Dublin and the United States, sometimes over one hundred thousand miles a year. As I was beyond traditional retirement age in Ireland (sixty-five years), I was on a five-year contract, which could not be renewed. As I approached the end of the fourth year, I was contacted by my old boss, Dr. Derek Raghavan, who had left the Cleveland Clinic to develop a new cancer institute in Charlotte, North Carolina. Derek wanted to develop survivorship services as part of the new institute and wondered if I might be interested. After some debate about the scope and scale of this initiative, I agreed to be the chair for a new Department of Supportive Oncology, which would include a Section of Palliative Medicine, integrating the concepts of supportive medicine and palliative medicine as had been proposed by a European Society for Medical Oncology position paper.[34] The new department would bring together all of the supportive care services for cancer patients in a single administrative entity, with multiple geographical locations potentially throughout both North and South Carolina.

THE ROAD AHEAD

The Department of Supportive Oncology is now three years old. In addition to Palliative Medicine, it includes sections of Oncology Nutrition, Cancer Rehabilitation, Survivorship, Senior Oncology, Integrative Oncology, and Navigation. We are also developing a Clinical Research Section to evaluate outcomes and investigate common complications of cancer and cancer treatments. Currently all our activities are outpatient. We have developed educational activities with two programs: the fellowship in medical oncology and the internal medicine residency. These also include a weekly supportive oncology department grand rounds and research meeting. More recently, we have created fellowships for training in supportive oncology, palliative medicine, psycho-oncology, and cancer rehabilitation.

We continue to grow rapidly in patient volumes. The most clinically active are palliative medicine, integrative oncology, and psycho-oncology. Cancer rehabilitation is close behind; the newer areas of senior oncology and survivorship (including cardio-oncology) are poised for growth. Typically, a new department will take five to seven years before it is mature, but we are well on the way, even as we face the challenge of dealing with the COVID-19 pandemic.[35]

PALLIATIVE MEDICINE MAINSTREAMED

In the wider medical community, it is fascinating to see that many of the ground rules of palliative medicine are now part of the fabric of modern medicine. These, in no particular order, include putting the patient first; better symptom control; a care team and multidisciplinary care; better design of health care facilities, including healing spaces; care for staff; continuity of care between the hospital and community; improved communication skills with patient and family; coordination of care and navigation; psychosocial care; and greater concern for the dying. These reflect a major cultural shift in medicine; they are to be welcomed. I find that oncologists, surgeons, and others are now receptive to palliative medicine (and the emerging area of supportive oncology). In previous years, suspicion and downright hostility was not unusual, since the goal of medicine was seen principally as resistance to death. Now the future looks bright. I have every confidence that, within a decade, every major cancer center in the United States will have a supportive oncology structure similar to the one in Charlotte. The patient demand is there, and the medical culture has adjusted to accept that modern cancer care should be whole-person care: treating the patient, not just the tumor.

Many challenges face medicine in general and palliative medicine in particular, but I have found in this career a lifetime of challenge—in terms of both obstacles to confront and opportunities to engage, professional and personal, both occasional and long-standing. There will probably always be a tension between exceptional health care and the exigencies of finances, between physicians and administrators, between patient expectations and physicians' abilities, between resources and dreams. There will probably always be these tensions, but they can be creative too. Cicely Saunders taught us that much, and I hope that this retrospect has continued in that vein, as I, too, have faced my share of challenges, with some battles lost and others won but always with the conviction that this is a vocation worth championing because of the opportunities it creates to embolden our patients and palliate their—*our*—inevitable pain.

NOTES

1. Flear, Walsh, and McCambridge 1977, 350.
2. Walsh 1977, 1071.
3. Walsh and Saunders 1984b.
4. Walsh and Leber 1982.
5. Walsh and West 1984; Walsh, Jackson, and Bowman 1982.
6. Lagman, Walsh, et al. 2007.
7. Walsh 1983a; Walsh, Bowman, and Jackson 1983; Walsh 1983b.
8. Walsh 1983c; Walsh and Cheater 1983; Walsh 1984b.
9. Walsh et al. 1994; Walsh 1994; Goldstein, Walsh, and Horvitz 1996.
10. Walsh and Saunders 1984a; Walsh 1984a.
11. Walsh 1985a.
12. Walsh 1985b.
13. Fanucchi et al. 1987.
14. Walsh 1989.
15. Smythe et al. 1992.
16. Walsh et al. 1994.
17. Walsh 1994.
18. Homsi et al. 2002.

19. Lagman and Walsh 2007; Lagman, Rivera, et al. 2007.
20. LeGrand et al. 2000.
21. Gallagher et al. 2001.
22. Walsh 1998; Davis et al. 2002.
23. Ahmedzai and Walsh 2000; Davis et al. 2001.
24. Walsh et al. 2000; Nelson and Walsh 2007.
25. Walsh 2004; Lagman and Walsh 2005; Davis et al. 2005.
26. Lagman and Walsh 2007; Lagman, Rivera, et al. 2007.
27. Lagman et al. 2011.
28. Lagman, Walsh, et al. 2007.
29. Goldstein, Walsh, and Horvitz 1996.
30. Walsh 2001.
31. Walsh et al. 2008.
32. Homsi et al. 2000; Zhukovsky, Walsh, and Tuason 2004; Davis et al. 2006; Yavuzsen et al. 2009.
33. Kenny et al. 2018; O'Donoghue et al. 2019.
34. Jordan et al. 2018.
35. Raghavan et al. 2020.

WORKS CITED

Ahmedzai, S., and D. Walsh. 2000. "Palliative Medicine and Modern Cancer Care." *Seminars in Oncology* 27 (1): 1–6.

Davis, M. P., D. Walsh, R. Lagman, and T. Yavuzsen. 2006. "Early Satiety in Cancer Patients: A Common and Important but Underrecognized Symptom." *Supportive Care in Cancer* 14 (7): 693–98.

Davis, M., D. Walsh, S. LeGrand, and R. Lagman. 2002. "End of Life Care: The Death of Palliative Medicine?" *Journal of Palliative Medicine* 5 (6): 813–14.

Davis, M., D. Walsh, S. B. LeGrand, R. L. Lagman, B. Harrison, and L. Rybicki. 2005. "The Financial Benefits of Acute Inpatient Palliative Medicine: An Inter-Institutional Comparative Analysis by All Patient Refined-Diagnosis Related Group and Case Mix Index." *Journal of Supportive Oncology* 3 (4): 1–4.

Davis, M., D. Walsh, K. Nelson, D. Konrad, and S. LeGrand. 2001. "The Business of Palliative Medicine: Management Metrics for an Acute Care Inpatient Unit." *American Journal of Hospice and Palliative Care* 18 (1): 26–29.

Fanucchi, M. P., T. D. Walsh, M. Fleischer, G. Lokos, L. Williams, C. Cassidy, D. Niedzwecki, and C. Young. 1987. "Phase I and Clinical Pharmacology Study of Trimetrexate Administered Weekly for Three Weeks." *Cancer Research* 47 (12): 3303–8.

Flear, B., T. D. Walsh, and H. J. McCambridge. 1977. "Actions of Cardiac Glycosides and Diuretics on Na-Pump Activity and Na-Permeability in Frog Ventricle Fibres." In "Proceedings of the British Cardiac Society." *British Heart Journal* 39 (3): 350.

Gallagher, L., M. Huston, D. Walsh, K. Nelson, and A. L. Steele. 2001. "Music Therapy in Palliative Medicine." *Supportive Care in Cancer* 9 (3): 156–61.

Goldstein, P., D. Walsh, and L. Horvitz. 1996. "The Cleveland Clinic Foundation Harry R. Horvitz Palliative Care Center." *Supportive Care in Cancer* 4 (5): 329–33.

Homsi, J., D. Walsh, K. Nelson, S. LeGrand, M. Davis, E. Khawam, and C. Nouneh. 2002. "The Impact of a Palliative Medicine Consultation Service in Medical Oncology." *Supportive Care in Cancer* 10 (4): 337–42.

Homsi, J., D. Walsh, R. Panta, R. Lagman, K. Nelson, D. Longworth. 2000. "Infectious Complications in Advanced Cancer." *Supportive Care in Cancer* 8 (6): 487–92.

Jordan, K., M. Aapro, S. Kaasa, C. I. Ripamonti, F. Scotte, F. Strasser, A. Young, E. Bruera, J. Herrstedt, D. Keefe, B. Laird, D. Walsh, J. Y. Douillard, and A. Cervantes. 2018. "European Society for Medical Oncology (ESMO) Position Paper on Supportive and Palliative Care." *Annals of Oncology* 29 (1): 36–43.

Kenny, C., O. Gilheaney, D. Walsh, and J. Regan. 2018. "Oropharyngeal Dysphagia Evaluation Tools in Adults with Solid Malignancies Outside the Head and Neck and Upper GI Tract: A Systematic Review." *Dysphagia* 33 (3): 303–20.

Lagman, R. L., N. Rivera, D. Walsh, S. LeGrand, and M. P. Davis. 2007. "Acute Inpatient Palliative Medicine in a Cancer Center: Clinical Problems and Medical Interventions—A Prospective Study." *American Journal of Hospice and Palliative Medicine* 24 (1): 20–28.

Lagman, R., and D. Walsh. 2005. "Integration of Palliative Medicine into Comprehensive Cancer Care." *Seminars in Oncology* 32 (2): 134–38.

———. 2007. "Acute Care Palliative Medicine: The Cleveland Model." *European Journal of Palliative Care* 14 (1): 17–20.

Lagman, R. L., D. Walsh, M. P. Davis, and B. Young. 2007. "All Patient Refined-Diagnostic Related Group and Case Mix Index in Acute Care Palliative Medicine." *Journal of Supportive Oncology* 5 (3): 145–49.

———. 2011. "The Business Model of Palliative Medicine Part 6: Clinical Operations in a Comprehensive Integrated Program." *American Journal of Hospice and Palliative Medicine* 28 (2): 75–81.

LeGrand, S., D. Walsh, K. Nelson, and D. Zhukovsky. 2000. "Development of a Fellowship Program in Palliative Medicine." *Journal of Pain and Symptom Management* 20 (5): 345–52.

Nelson, K., and D. Walsh. 2003. "The Business of Palliative Medicine Part 3: The Development of a Palliative Medicine Program in an Academic Medical Center." *American Journal of Hospice and Palliative Care* 20 (5): 345–52.

O'Donoghue, N., S. Shrotriya, A. Aktas, B. Hullihen, S. Ayvaz, B. Estfan, and D. Walsh. 2019. "Clinical Significance of Weight Changes at Diagnosis in Solid Tumors." *Supportive Care in Cancer* 27 (7): 2725–33.

Raghavan, D., E. S. Kim, S. J. Chai, K. Plate, E. Copelan, T. D. Walsh, S. Burri, J. Brown, and L. Musselwhite. 2020. "Levine Cancer Institute Approach to Pandemic Care of Patients with Cancer." *JCO Oncology Practice* 16 (6): 299–304.

Smythe, E., T. D. Walsh, K. Currie, P. Glare, and J. Schneider. 1992. "A Pilot Study, Review of the Literature, and Dosing Guidelines for Patient-Controlled Analgesia Using Subcutaneous Morphine Sulphate for Chronic Cancer Pain." *Palliative Medicine* 6 (3): 217–26.

Walsh, T. D. 1977. "Costochondritis." *New England Journal of Medicine* 297 (19): 1071.

———. 1983a. "Antidepressants in Chronic Pain." *Clinical Neuropharmacology* 6 (4): 271–95.

———. 1983b. "Measurement of Morphine: Clinical Pharmacokinetic Considerations During Chronic Administration." In *Modern Methods of Morphine Estimation*, edited by J. F. B. Stuart, 3–7. International Congress and Symposium 58. London: Academic Press and the Royal Society of Medicine.

———. 1983c. "Terminal Care: Pain Relief in Cancer." *Medicine in Practice* 1 (27): 684–91.

———. 1984a. "A Controlled Study of MST Continuous Tablets for Chronic Pain in Advanced Cancer." In *Advances in Morphine Therapy*, edited by E. Wilkes and J. Levy, 99–102. International Congress and Symposium 64. London: Royal Society of Medicine.

———. 1984b. "Oral Morphine in Chronic Cancer Pain." *Pain* 18 (1): 1–11.

———. 1985a. "Common Misunderstandings About the Use of Morphine for Chronic Pain in Advanced Cancer." *CA: A Cancer Journal for Clinicians* 35 (3): 164–69.

———. 1985b. "Symptom Control in Pain Patients." In *Management of Cancer Pain: Syllabus of a Postgraduate Course*, Memorial Sloan Kettering Cancer Center, November 14–16, 285–89.

———, ed. 1989. *Symptom Control*. Boston: Blackwell Scientific.

———. 1994. "Palliative Care: Management of the Patient with Advanced Cancer." *Seminars in Oncology* 21 (4): 100–106.

———. 1998. "The Medicare Hospice Benefit: A Critique from Palliative Medicine." *Palliative Medicine* 1 (2): 147–49.

———. 2001. "The Harry R. Horvitz Center for Palliative Medicine (1987–1999): Development of a Novel Comprehensive Integrated Program." *American Journal of Hospice and Palliative Care* 18 (4): 239–50.

————. 2004. "The Business of Palliative Medicine—Part 4: Potential Impact of an Acute-Care Palliative Medicine Inpatient Unit in a Tertiary Care Cancer Center." *American Journal of Hospice and Palliative Care* 21 (3): 217–21.

————, ed. 2008. *Palliative Medicine*. Philadelphia: W. B. Saunders.

Walsh, T. D., K. B. Bowman, and G. P. Jackson. 1983. "Dietary Intake of Advanced Cancer Patients." *Journal of Human Nutrition: Applied Nutrition* 37 (A): 41–45.

Walsh, T. D., and F. M. Cheater. 1983. "Use of Morphine for Cancer Pain." *Pharmaceutical Journal* 10 (January): 525–27.

Walsh, D., M. Doona, M. Molnar, and V. Lipnickey. 2000. "Symptom Control in Advanced Cancer: Important Drugs and Routes of Administration." *Seminars in Oncology* 27 (1): 69–83.

Walsh, T. D., W. R. Gombeski, P. Goldstein, D. Hayes, and M. Armour. 1994. "Managing a Palliative Oncology Program: The Role of a Business Plan." *Journal of Pain and Symptom Management* 9 (2): 109–18.

Walsh, T. D., G. P. Jackson, and K. B. Bowman. 1982. "Dietary Intake of Advanced Cancer Patients." *Proceedings of the Nutrition Society* 41 (3): 96A.

Walsh, T. D., and B. Leber. 1982. "Measurement of Chronic Pain: Visual Analogue Scales and Mcgill-Melzack Pain Questionnaire Compared." In *Proceedings of the Third World Congress on Pain*, edited by J. J. Bonica, U. Lindblom, and A. Iggo, 897–99. Vol. 5 of *Advances in Pain Research and Therapy*. New York: Raven Press.

Walsh, T. D., and C. M. Saunders. 1984a. "Depression in Advanced Cancer." *The Treatment of Depression in General Practice*, Bulletin 12.

————. 1984b. "Hospice Care: The Treatment of Pain in Advanced Cancer." In *Pain in the Cancer Patient: Pathogenesis, Diagnosis and Therapy*, edited by M. Zimmermann, P. Drings, and G. Wagner, 201–11. Recent Results in Cancer Research 89. Berlin: Springer-Verlag.

Walsh, T. D., and T. S. West. 1984. "Malignant Ureteric Obstruction Relieved by Dexamethasone." *Postgraduate Medical Journal* 60 (704): 437–38.

Yavuzsen, T., D. Walsh, M. P. Davis, T. Jin, S. LeGrand, R. Lagman, J. Kirkova, L. Bicanovsky, B. Estfan, B. Cheema, and A. Haddad. 2009. "Components of the Anorexia-Cachexia Syndrome: Gastrointestinal Symptom Correlates of Cancer Anorexia." *Supportive Care in Cancer* 17 (12): 1531–42.

Zhukovsky, D., D. Walsh, and L. Tuason. 2004. "Communication in Palliative Medicine: Use of a Problem List for Multidisciplinary Care." *American Journal of Hospice and Palliative Care* 21 (5): 365–71.

Palliative Care

Pain and Suffering

CHAPTER 5

Time to Death

Chronos, Kairos, *and the "Longest Distance Between Two Poles"*

Joseph J. Fins

TIME TRAVEL

Tennessee Williams's *The Glass Menagerie* premiered in Chicago in 1944 amidst the brutality of the Battle of the Bulge and the horrors of war in Europe and the Pacific.[1] As the play opens, the narrator, Tom, orients the audience to the nature of the performance. He explains, "The play is memory. Being a memory play, it is dimly lighted, it is sentimental, it is not realistic." He promises to "turn back time" to "that quaint period, the thirties, when the huge middle class of America was matriculating in a school for the blind." Tom's opening monologue is a retrospective, a looking back on our naïveté, our willingness to embrace "deceptive rainbows" even as the world marched toward fascism and world war. The performance to follow is "truth in the pleasant guise of illusion." It isn't until the play's conclusion that he reveals that the illusion is about time. Responding to his overbearing mother, who wants him to shoot for the stars, Tom retorts, "I didn't go to the moon. I went much further—for time is the longest distance between two poles."

Tom's quip is perhaps the most famous line from the *Menagerie*. It is invoked often to convey the power of time to frame, inform, and distort our narratives. Tom reminds us, in a play that yearns for a forgone past and looks to an elusive future, that time is a more compelling variable than how far one has come or how much farther one has to travel. Those journeys are subservient to how they are recalled and understood temporally and not merely a measure of the distance traveled. To see the voyage as simply the distance between two poles is to miss the depth or true length of the journey. Indeed, to reduce it to a measurement is to engage in a sort of reductionism that trivializes the plot.

What does this have to do with palliative care? I believe a similar illusion informs how we think about pedagogy and palliation. We tend to construct truths that are equally quaint. We think of the distance between poles of wellness and illness and fail to realize that the true distance traversed is more temporal than spatial. When we create these simplistic heuristics, we indulge in an illusion of certainty that obscures the confusion and indeterminacy that only temporality can convey.

Consider the ubiquitous phrase "at life's end," which graces the palliative care literature to discuss the ethical and clinical choices in palliative care. In fact, the fragment is part of the subtitle of my book, *A Palliative Ethic of Care: Clinical Wisdom at Life's End.*[2] But as I reflect on these words, and a title scripted over a decade ago, I feel compelled to assess critically the phrase. And when doing so I must confess a degree of naïveté in creating my own "deceptive rainbow."

The phrase seems to simplify things, as if writing of life's end from the other side. That is, retrospectively, from the perspective of knowing that life was at its end. With this perspective comes the certain confidence of hindsight, and with the unfailing prediction that a patient has arrived at a destination, that life's journey is complete or will soon be. The mystery, the undulations that characterize a disease trajectory (much less life), is smoothed out by rhetoric. Through our discourse we imply more knowledge than we really possess. While we know it will end, we don't know how and when. There is almost always more complexity than is subsumed by that seemingly simple phrase, "at life's end."

When we divide the world this way, we fall into a false dichotomy between curative efforts and palliative care. Though we might falsely imagine there is a bright line distinction between these two spheres, the reality is that most care tends to be blended, a mosaic. The reality is that many cancer-directed therapies are palliative rather than curative. A wise oncologist delivering her ministrations might appreciate that while she treats with a curative intent, the science says what she is doing is palliative. But can this always be recognized, given the power of self-delusion and the desire not to disappoint the expectant patient?

This degree of nuance can be especially challenging when trying to teach end-of-life care. Educators simplify things and adopt a binary framework. It is an understandable pedagogical strategy. Once life's trajectory has played out, we can confidently prescribe our ministrations without fear of misjudgment. The phrase suggests that, while a curative approach might have been better suited for the ongoing journey, a palliative stance is more appropriate when the end is in sight. With this clarity, one can be prescriptive and provide care during a difficult time.

But how patients die is more complicated than our rhetorical devices. It is never so simple. As Kierkegaard famously noted, life is lived forward and understood backward.[3] So, too, it is in death, which can sometimes only be apprehended in retrospect.

Nevertheless, palliative care education persists in invoking this approach with the notion of what clinicians should do at life's end, as if we had a biomarker for impending death. While this rhetorical device is less problematic when patients are imminently dying, it becomes a challenge when the goal is to move palliative care upstream. How does a clinician know when to make the transition from curative to palliative care? How does the balance of utility and futility[4] coalesce into a diagnostic, or better yet prognostic, framework to suggest that an inflection point has been reached?

Except in the most obvious of cases, there will be uncertainty. And when there is uncertainty, how does the specter of death—real or imagined—inform choices and actions by patients, families, and clinicians? When death is foretold, to invoke the title of Nicholas Christakis's elegant volume on prognosis,[5] does it make it more likely? Or does the uncertainty lead to preemption? Consider the mantra of those who advance aid-in-dying so as to control the "timing and manner" of one's death, a phrase invoked in *Washington v. Glucksberg* (521 US 702 [1997]), the Supreme Court case that litigated the constitutional right to assisted suicide. The data from Oregon, where assisted suicide has been decriminalized, suggest that, while physician-assisted suicide provides pain relief for some, the vast majority of those who avail themselves of this option do so because of uncertainty and angst about the future, about what comes next.[6]

And what happens when our predictions are wrong? We often speak of a failure to thrive. But what of a failure to die?[7] What happens when death is eluded by good care, or good fortune, when our prognoses fall short in accuracy and patients live longer than expected? Or when public policy misconstrues how long it takes to die? Consider the Medicare Hospice Benefit, which stipulates a six-month prognosis for eligibility and the response of physicians and hospice administrators who delay referrals lest they be subject to administrative audit and fiscal claw-backs when a patient, in the crassest of terms, lives too long and, consequently, outlives a benefit [42 C.F.R. § 418.202(e)]?[8]

All of these questions relate to questions of judgment and time.

A RETROSPECTIVE

As would be appropriate, time has afforded me the opportunity to ask these questions and reflect back on a period of my life—and work—dominated by palliative care. For the last twenty years, my scholarly focus has increasingly been on severe brain injury and disorders of consciousness.[9] While I have introduced the notion of neuro-palliative care for these patients,[10] for the most part my scholarship in neuroethics and severe brain injury has displaced my work in mainstream palliative care, which had been my academic focus for the previous decade and a half. While I continue to do clinical ethics and chair a hospital ethics committee, and while I encounter death and dying on a daily basis, I sit at arm's length from the academic work that is taking place in the field. As such, I have been more an observer than a participant in its evolution and how it has been institutionalized over the past couple of decades.

While this standardization is generally for the good and was inevitable as one generation of scholars bequeathed their work to the next, the protocolization of palliative care has not been without its costs and liabilities. One of those costs has been to lose sight of individual narratives and our sense of time, as patients and families make their transition from wellness to illness and death. As the late writer Paul Cowan wrote in the *Village Voice*, as he was dying of leukemia, "the world is divided between the sick and the not yet sick."[11]

The challenge is that these transitions cannot be known in advance. They can only be apprehended in retrospect. But as my generation of physician-scholars sought to legitimize palliative care amidst an overwhelmingly curative ethos that then, and now, infused medical practice, we needed somehow to find a way to write, teach, and practice palliative care. We needed an anchor to make sense of the transitions and the change in goals of care from "curing to caring," as the saying went at the time. So we worked backward from death, both clinically and pedagogically, using that mantra as our touchstone.

In the mid-1990s, we saw this in the efforts of the Open Society Institute's *Project on Death in America* (PDIA),[12] the highly influential effort of financier George Soros. At least *rhetorically*, it was not about an effort to improve palliative care in America. Rather, true to its name, its goal was to "transform the culture of death and dying in America."[13] Moving from the realm of academics and think tanks to the popular culture, the debate during that era was about physician-assisted suicide, later euphemistically rephrased to "medical aid-in-dying." At least as I see it, the nomenclature of the death-and-dying movement was focused on the end game and not the process that led to our leaving this mortal coil.

In hospital life during that period of time, palliative care was reduced to whether or not an eager house officer had "gotten" a DNR, or do-not-resuscitate order. This was a plan for the last fifteen minutes of a patient's life and nothing more. The focus was more on the destination and less about the journey. I remember, with great self-satisfaction, my own successes as a house officer obtaining a DNR order where others had failed and thinking that I had provided for a good death. While I might have protected the patient—and the family—from what would have most likely been a futile assault on their body and personhood, I was remarkably unaware of broader patient and family needs as they made the journey from serious to terminal illness. The focus was on death and not so much on dying.

This may have been a consequence of my generation's need to make sense of the idiosyncrasy of a field that was new and cobbled together from a range of disciplines.[14] We needed end points and clarity. Death was the ultimate outcome measure that helped to orient the work. Lest we forget, in the 1990s there were no palliative care boards. The field was looking for legitimacy and cohesion. It was eclectic and composed of clinicians from a broad range of practice. The leading lights in the field who served as mentors to my generation were neurologists and neuro-oncologists turned palliative care experts who cared for cancer patients; geriatricians; pain-management specialists in anesthesia and pharmacology; and psycho-oncologists: psychiatrists and psychologists who cared for terminally ill cancer patients. Given this diversity of disciplines, a common focus was needed, and so death became our lodestar.

It was an exciting time for those of us who were making a professional journey into something new and making it up along the way. I wistfully remember
my time as a PDIA faculty scholar and how, as my cohort came together, we
struggled to make sense of how we arrived there and later where this emerging field was headed.

One vivid memory I have was of our initial gathering at a rustic retreat
in Pictou, Nova Scotia. We sat together in a screened porch and shared our
personal narratives, trying to explain why we had all veered off the path and
decided to do palliative care.

As we went around our little circle of friends, we told our stories. Lost
parents, a sibling who died too young, patients who suffered and were lost, as
well as other formative tragedies that left stigmata on our souls. When it was
my turn, I was surprised by what I said. It was unplanned, and, if I had been
more on guard, I might have spoken of a patient for whom I had cared during
medical school or residency. But to my surprise I spoke of my grandmother,
who had severe angina, and how she had suffered. In the 1960s, there wasn't
much to do for her. She popped nitroglycerin pills when she walked about
her Florida apartment and took solace from a large green oxygen tank in the
corner of her bedroom. She was a proud self-made woman from Lithuania.
Brave and strong. But I saw how the angina furrowed her brow; it broke my
little boy's heart. I loved her so, because my own mom adored her. So it was
a filial thing, and it upset me more than I knew.

As we reflected on our paths in the cool breeze of an August afternoon, I
spoke of my interest in cardiology in high school. The dissection in my base-
ment of a cow's heart, which my mother had gotten from the local butcher.
How I volunteered in my local emergency room and taught myself how to
read cardiograms by reading Dubin's text,[15] a guide used by generations of
medical students to learn the rudiments of electrocardiography. Later still, I
worked with a pediatric cardiologist in college doing early work on the ability
of nuclear magnetic resonance—a precursor to modern *f*MRI imaging—to
identify cardiac infarctions in laboratory animals. It was exciting work.

But as I studied the humanities in college and went to medical school, the
need to attend to human pain and suffering drew me in. Yes, cardiology had
made strides. If my grandmother had survived a few more years, she would
have found relief—perhaps in the guise of a beta blocker, angioplasty, or
bypass surgery—but what of those who didn't, what of those patients who
needed the solace and comfort of palliation? For others, the benefit of all

these emergent technologies had run their course. They found themselves *at life's end* even if their doctors didn't yet appreciate that the end was nigh.

It was a remarkable conversation that afternoon. While each of us had a different story with a distinct set of characters, each of us had had similar trajectories to palliative care. For the most part, our interests were not born of technical fascination with the physiology of dying or the pharmacology of pain management. We migrated into what would become palliative care because of the power of narratives to transform our lives.

I have indulged in this autobiographical digression because each of us of that generation of palliative care became cultural change agents, as the PDIA envisioned us to be,[16] and had an unscripted and unexpected entry into palliative care. As similar as our journeys were, when we heard each other's stories, each of us experienced them as personal and idiosyncratic. We weren't following a well-worn path; we "learned by doing," to invoke a Deweyan notion.[17] And, most critically, we arrived in the space in our own time. It was hardly preordained or fated.

These experiences informed how we reflected upon our patients' journeys. But not in the way we might have been expected. Instead of celebrating our idiosyncratic journeys, we recoiled against their randomness and sought intellectually to impose order on our field and its nascent structure. Training programs and fellowships and curricula were established.[18] Efforts to create board certification were undertaken and achieved. Outcomes took precedence over process.[19] What had been something of a cottage industry was formalized and institutionalized.

Much good has followed from these developments. This is probably the way it should be as the sociology of fields emerge, evolve, and become established. The energy of the founding generations morphs into organizational structures that disseminate new knowledge and legitimate the field's academic and clinical enterprise. There is nothing unusual about this process of evolution, and we are all the better for it.[20]

But as we acknowledge what has been gained through this process, it is also important to register what has been lost with the advent of institutionalization and choices made by institutions. The field has become more about protocols than personalities and patient particularities. While there is less idiosyncrasy, so, too, there is a prescriptive disregard of particularities and of the power of patient narratives to inform empathic response. This outcome is especially ironic, given the origins of palliative care and the centrality of narrative to those who helped found the field. Here I think of Dame Cicely Saunders, Kathleen Foley, Richard Payne, Eduardo Bruera, Russell Portenoy—and younger colleagues from my own generational cohort.

TIME, NARRATIVE, AND BRAIN INJURY

Narrative and time are inextricably linked. A good story needs time to develop and redound onto itself. Time allows for reflection and memory, the motivating aesthetic of *The Glass Menagerie*. To compress a story is to rob it of its power to inform and transform. The impatient reader who consults a synopsis misses the experience of accompanying a character through a play or novel. CliffsNotes just won't do.

The same is true for patient narratives. If life imitates fiction, then paring down patient narratives to the "essentials" is to disregard how the twists and turns in their stories informed their lives and will shape their deaths. At best, the clinician who acts as an expeditious editor will deprive herself of the aesthetic richness of thick descriptions. At worst, it can lead to an omission that veers toward iatrogenesis, doctor-induced harm. If time *is* the longest distance between two points, its compression can have dire consequences.

A mathematical illustration, for those who are so inclined, follows in the next couple of paragraphs. If you want to skip the math and get back to the narrative, feel free to skip the next two paragraphs . . .

Mathematically, this can be represented as $P = dD/dT$, where P is prognosis, D is diagnosis, and T is time. In the aggregate, this differential equation will plot the *change* of a patient's diagnosis or condition over time. The curve depicted by the equation will become the patient's trajectory.

However, if time, the denominator of this differential, is compressed, the curve resulting from this differential equation will be skewed. What would normally happen *over time* will be accelerated. At the extreme, if time were eliminated completely, if time were *totally compressed*, then the patient's current diagnosis would also become his prognosis. There would be no change. It would all be in the moment. What should be a curve would become a point representing the present. Any discussion of prognosis over time would become moot because the patient's current state would be all there was. There would be no past or future. Without time, the patient's *current* condition would become the *calculus* of all decisions. Eliminating the influence of time, there would be no need to think ahead because the present would be all that matters. While this could make things simpler, it could also preclude salubrious changes that might occur over time. In some scenarios it might preclude recovery.

Consider the case of the patient who is admitted to the hospital unconscious following a severe traumatic brain injury. The family is asked to make a decision about curative or palliative care. They see their unconscious loved one and project the patient's current state forward assuming that her current status will persist. The situation seems grave, and the clinicians recommend that "aggressive" treatment not be pursued to protect the patient from a dire future. A decision is made to withhold or withdraw life-sustaining therapy, and the patient expires.

This is troubling. While the loss of consciousness can be life-threatening, it is not invariably so. By preempting the patient's future, by compressing time, the doctors have precluded alternate outcomes that they could not apprehend because they did not, could not, have perfect knowledge. At that juncture in the patient's course, they were of course correct, but only because they had compressed time. They had reduced the patient's trajectory to the present, precluding the future. This compression of time meant that what might have been will never be. It falsely falls prey to the false dichotomy between care and cure that was critiqued earlier on.

My vignette is more than a hypothetical parable to elaborate my argument. It is routine practice. A recent study reported that 70.2 percent of the 31.7 percent in-hospital mortality for disorders of consciousness stemmed from a decision to withdraw life-sustaining therapy, for example, to remove a patient from a ventilator.[21] Put another way, seven out of ten patients who die from severe brain injury do not die because nature has taken its course but rather due to a decision to stop treatment. While some of those patients would have invariably died, many would not have, but they are equally dead because time was compressed and their future was precluded.

There are several reasons why this practice pattern persists. The first is the culture of death and dying in America. Simply to articulate an argument that I have elaborated at great length in *Rights Come to Mind* and elsewhere,[22] the right to die in America was established in the setting of severe brain injury and particularly the vegetative state. From *Quinlan* to *Cruzan* to *Schiavo*, the inevitable futility of these brain states became the moral warrant to establish the right to die. In his landmark decision in *Quinlan*, Chief Judge Richard

Hughes of the New Jersey Supreme Court justified the removal of Ms. Quinlan's ventilator based on the unlikely prospect of the return of "any semblance
of cognitive or sapient life" (*In re Quinlan*, 70 N.J. 10, 355 A.2d 647 [NJ 1976]).

This presumption of qualitative futility, which began in the vegetative state,
was generalized to other disorders of consciousness with which it may be confused. Consider the advice of Wijdicks and Rabinstein, who counsel clinicians
to temper their hopes for patients in the comatose state: "The attending physician of a patient with a devastating neurologic illness will have to come to
terms with the futility of care.... Those families who are unconvinced should
be explicitly told they should have markedly diminished expectations for what
intensive care can accomplish and that withdrawal of life support or abstain-
ing from performing complex interventions is more commensurate with the
neurologic status."[23] Such advice further compresses time and limits outcomes
because the advice is for patients in a *comatose state*, which is itself time-limited
and generally has a duration of two weeks or less, unless it is medically prolonged. At that point, patients either regain consciousness or move on to the
vegetative or minimally conscious state. The challenge with this prescriptive
advice is that it has compressed the full prognostic possibilities of a patient's
course into the compressed confines of the initial presentation.

There is another misconstrual about time that plays into these precipitous
compressions and that is an error in analogic reasoning about the loss of consciousness. In routine medical practice, most "do not attempt resuscitation"
(DNAR) orders are consented to by family members acting as surrogates
when the patient loses capacity because of a medical deterioration.[24] This can
be the result of advancing cancer or heart disease or dementia. The patient's
loss of consciousness or more generally decisional capacity, and with it the lost
potential for interpersonal engagement, is viewed as a harbinger of impending
death. These patients have a downward trajectory. Their disease has progressed
to the point that they have lost consciousness. But the loss of consciousness
that occurs with severe brain injury is potentially something quite distinct.
Their loss of consciousness, while it could lead to death, could also be the
beginning of a recovery process.[25] Again, this is a question of temporal perception. Is the patient coming or going?

Recent developments in how neurology has named disorders of consciousness has further pointed to the centrality of time in how we think about
these patients. In September 2018, the American Academy of Neurology
(AAN), the American College of Rehabilitation Medicine (ACRM), and

the National Institute on Disability, Independent Living, and Rehabilitation Research (NIDILRR) published a systematic, evidence-based review[26] and a new practice guideline[27] on the care of patients with disorders of consciousness. While there is much to discuss about the ethical, palliative, and legal implications of this work,[28] for our purposes the key development was the *redesignation* of the permanent vegetative state to the chronic vegetative state. Based on their review of the biology and epidemiology of the permanent vegetative state, these experts maintained that 20 percent of patients thought to be permanently vegetative could regain consciousness, prompting the change from permanent to chronic.

In many ways, this change was a vindication of the original analysis of Bryan Jennett and Fred Plum in their 1972 landmark paper in the *Lancet*, where they first described the vegetative state and their musings on time.[29] Jennett was the Scottish neurosurgeon who created the Glasgow Coma and Outcome Scales. Plum was an American neurologist who described the "locked-in state" and served as chair of neurology at Cornell, where he was my teacher and, later, colleague. In their paper, they detail how they came up with the name "*persistent* vegetative state."

Elsewhere I have explained why they chose "vegetative" for what they described as a state of wakeful unresponsiveness.[30] Here I want to focus on why their choice to describe this brain state as "persistent" matters. In describing the vegetative state as persistent, they were concerned about time and how to capture the duration of the brain state. They wanted to be accurate in the use of any modifier. "Persistent" was chosen as an adjective so as not to imply permanence and to express their uncertainty about the likelihood of permanent unconsciousness.

Clearly focused on temporal issues, Jennett and Plum explained their rationale: "Certainly we are concerned to identify an irrevocable state, although the criteria needed to establish that prediction reliably have still to be confirmed. Until then 'persistent' is safer than '*permanent*' or '*irreversible*'; but *prolonged* is not strong enough, and unless it is quantified it is meaningless."[31] Theirs is a remarkably careful analysis of the temporal uncertainty attendant on the vegetative state. Their explication suggests that, instead of compressing time, they did *precisely the opposite* when they chose "persistent" versus "permanent" versus "irreversible."

Instead of *compressing* time, Jennett and Plum were attentive to their relative ignorance as they worked on the cutting edge of neurology circa 1972.

They wanted to leave open the possibility of evolving, dynamic brain states and not preclude outcomes that might yet occur and that they could only anticipate.[32] In addition to the logical rigor of their deliberations, it could also be said that they brought temporal humility to their analysis. So given their doubts and lack of temporal data, they left the prognosis associated with this brain state more open-ended. And history has been kind to them, even if it took a detour.[33]

Despite Jennett and Plum's hesitancy about designating the vegetative state as permanent, that is what happened two decades later. The 1994 Multi-Society Task Force Report on the Vegetative State subsequently distinguished the persistent from the permanent vegetative state. As per this classification, the vegetative state became persistent after a month's duration and permanent three months after anoxic injury or twelve months after traumatic injury.[34] This classification scheme *persisted* until it was revised in 2018 with the redesignation of "permanent" as "chronic."[35] This revision acknowledged that some patients will recover above the vegetative state after alleged permanence had set in, a validation of Jennett and Plum's original formulation nearly a half century earlier.[36]

CHRONOS AND KAIROS

How did Jennett and Plum get it right? Before CT scans and functional neuroimaging and without decades of clinical observations to aid them, how did they know to limit their claims? That is, how did they convey that the vegetative would have a long duration, without claiming that it would inevitably be so? How did they know it was *not the right time* to make the leap to permanence, a nosological change that was made in 1994 only to be reversed in 2018 by contravening data?

Jennett and Plum's prudence is a feat to behold. I believe that, like the name "vegetative," which goes back to Aristotle's *De Anima*,[37] their decision to choose "persistent" over "permanent" goes back to the Greeks. In ancient Greek, there are two words for time, *chronos* and *kairos*, as explained by the late Professor John E. Smith of Yale University in an exceptional essay published in the *Monist* in 1969.[38]

As Smith enumerates, *chronos* is the notion of time with which we are most familiar. It is a quantitative measure that captures how long something takes, how much longer we have to go, the age or duration of something. It is useful to track our travel times, all the more so when we set a chronometer on our watch. When we talk of the passage of time, we mean *chronos*.

Kairos or timeliness, on the other hand, is qualitatively different. It measures nothing but takes the measure of an occasion. While *chronos* tells us time to destination, *kairos* tells us whether it is an opportune time to make that trip. This could be something as mundane as whether the weather should prompt a postponement. Or, if the trip were an important pilgrimage, whether or not the sojourner was ready to make the journey. It places the journey into a broader context and speaks to the timing of the trip or the quality of the voyage. In this way, *kairos* describes the timeliness of an event.

Returning to the musings of Jennett and Plum,[39] they had a sense of the duration of the vegetative state (*chronos*), but they weren't sure it was an opportune time to say so (*kairos*). They recognized, at least implicitly, that *chronos* in the absence of *kairos* is not a full measure of our time. Even as subsequent scholars stepped into the fray in 1994,[40] only to be reversed in 2018,[41] Jennett and Plum waited. *Kairos* was not on their side. It was not the time to be more definitive, and so they waited. Medicine and neurology would have to wait for the right time.

Sadly, neither Jennett nor Plum lived to see the redesignation of the permanent vegetative state. But their legacy transcends the naming of the vegetative state and informs broader questions about palliative care. Their reticence suggests that, for important decisions that involve time and timing, *chronos* alone is insufficient for tempered decisions. While we need a sense of duration, or a shared chronology, to start life-altering discussions, that information takes us only so far. *Kairos* must also enter the equation to provide depth and context.

When clinicians talk about life expectancy or say a patient is at life's end, they are invoking a shallow conception of time. They are conceptualizing time as *chronos* without adequately asking questions of meaning, narrative, and context, which raise deeper questions about whether it is a *particular patient's time to die.*

Chronos as exemplified through prognosis cannot accommodate the personal. Only *kairos* can speak to a right moment, a turning point that presents an opportunity for action. Before this juncture, a decision is too early. Afterward, it is too late. As Smith reminds us, what *kairos* captures is a "special temporal position."[42] In a subsequent essay, he makes an explicit etymological link between *kairos* and rhetoric, pointing to the importance of narrative to this dimension of time.[43]

This may seem a semantic distinction, but it is not only that. An overreliance on *chronos* without regard to *kairos* leads to formulaic approaches to palliative care and medical education that displace the patient's story. An overreliance on *chronos* displaces the individual's narrative, which is essential for clinical deliberation and determining how a patient will die. Only *kairos* provides this sense of timing, a right time for something to occur. Yes, a patient has very advanced metastatic disease. Yes, *chronos* is not on their side. But what if they still have a life project to complete or a family event to attend? What if the patient is a parent with young children who feels compelled to press on? Their time may be up, but they don't see it that way.

SOLID GOLD WATCHES

Sometimes the poet knows what the scientist comes to understand.[44] And so it was with Tennessee Williams, whose *The Glass Menagerie* began our foray into time and whose less well-known *The Last of My Solid Gold Watches* will help us draw this essay to a conclusion.[45] I write "conclusion" advisedly, as I hope that it is the proper time for me to end this piece, with all due respect to a developed sense of *kairos*.

Williams, as *The Glass Menagerie* revealed, was preoccupied by time and saw it as more than the distance between two points. In *Gold Watches*—which could be seen as a companion piece to the *Menagerie*—we see glimmers of his appreciation of *kairos*, of that which fills in the length between those two points and provides depth to distance. The story takes place in a hotel room in the sweltering Mississippi Delta. A grizzled old shoe salesman reminisces about the past glories of plying his trade. Alternately, he meets a younger salesman at the start of his career and an African American porter who has worked at the hotel for decades.

Mr. Charlie, a character modeled upon Williams's father, who also sold shoes in the Delta, reminds his younger colleague, "When you arrive at my age—which is seventy-eight—you have a perspective of time on earth that astounds you!" He recounts how all his friends are dying, one carrying a casket, one struck by lightning, and yet another who had a stroke and caught fire when the cigar dangling out of his mouth caused a fire. It is one tale of woe after another. He tells the younger man, "Maybe you don't know it—but all of us ole-timers, Bob, are disappearin' *fast*! We all gotta quit th' road one time or another. Me, I reckon I'm pretty near the last of th' Delta drummers!"

Now ruminating more than reflecting, the older man explains, "Mortality, that was the trouble! Some people think that millions now living are never going to *die*. I don't think that—I think it's a misapprehension not borne out by the facts." A celebrated salesman, who has won fifteen gold watches for his accomplishments, he laments—"The world I knew is gone—gone—gone with the wind! My pockets are full of watches which tell me that my time's just about over!" The symbolism is an overt nod to *chronos* and the passage of time.

Later, as he speaks alone to the hotel porter, his tone shifts, as his sense of time deepens, and there is remorse over how his world, *their* world, has changed. The porter, "solemnly nodding," reminds Mr. Charlie, "The graveyard is crowded with folks we knew, Mistuh Charlie. It's mighty late in the day."

Then there is the recognition that time isn't all what it seems to be. It is more than *chronos*; there is also *kairos*. The two old men realize that it is later than they both think. As Mr. Charlie crosses over to the window, he tells his old acquaintance, "It ain't even late in the day any more—[*He throws up the blind*] It's NIGHT! [The space of the window is black]." And later, "softly, with a wise old smile," the porter replies, "Yes, suh. . . . *Night*, Mistuh Charlie!"

My colleague Barrie Huberman recently told me that "time leaves room for things to happen."[46] And so it does in this final scene. Both men, separated by race and class in a distant time, share a moment of reflection about time. After all their years together in the segregated South, they find themselves in the same time and place, facing mortality with insight and a "wise old smile" from an unexpected corner. It is an artful and beautiful moment, which, to this reader's eye, is the essence of palliation: the comfort that comes with knowing that time has passed and that one's time has come. Simply put, Williams has captured time in its fullest, the unification of both *chronos* and *kairos*. We should aspire to such artistry in our care of patients, as we help them traverse the longest distance between two poles.

NOTES

1. Williams 1999.
2. Fins 2006.
3. Kierkegaard 2003, from the Berlin 1843 journal; Fins 2017a.
4. Callahan 1994.
5. Christakis 2000.
6. Fins 2014; Fins and Morrissey 2018.
7. Fins 2002.

8. Fins 2017b.

9. Fins 2015.

10. Fins 2008; Fins and Pohl 2015; Fins and Master 2017.

11. Cowan 1988.

12. Aulino and Foley 2001.

13. McGlinchey 2004.

14. Fins 1999.

15. Dubin 1973.

16. McGlinchey 2004.

17. Dewey 1988, 1–62.

18. Morrison et al. 2018.

19. National Quality Forum 2006.

20. Swensen et al. 2010.

21. Turgeon et al. 2011.

22. Fins 2015; Fins and Plum 2004.

23. Wijdicks and Rabinstein 2007.

24. Fins et al. 1999.

25. Fins 2007, 2019a.

26. Giacino et al. 2018a.

27. Ibid.

28. Fins and Bernat 2018; Fins 2019c.

29. Jennett and Plum 1972.

30. Adams and Fins 2017; Fins 2019c.

31. Jennett and Plum 1972.

32. Fins and Schiff 2017.

33. Fins 2019b.

34. Multi-Society Task Force on PVS 1994a, 1994b.

35. Giacino et al. 2018b.

36. Jennett and Plum 1972.

37. Adams and Fins 2017.

38. Smith 1969.

39. Jennett and Plum 1972.

40. Fins and Schiff 2017.

41. Giacino et al. 2018b.

42. Smith 1969.

43. Smith 2002.

44. Fins 2020.

45. Williams 1966.

46. B. Huberman, personal communication with the author, August 2019.

WORKS CITED

Adams, Z. M., and J. J. Fins. 2017. "The Historical Origins of the Vegetative State: Received Wisdom and the Utility of the Text." *Journal of the History of the Neurosciences* 26 (2): 140–53.

Aulino, F., and K. Foley. 2001. "The Project on Death in America." *Journal of the Royal Society of Medicine* 94 (9): 492–95.

Callahan, D. 1994. "Necessity, Futility, and the Good Society." *Journal of the American Geriatrics Society* 42 (8): 866–67.

Christakis, N. A. 2000. *Death Foretold: Prophecy and Prognosis in Medical Care*. Chicago: University of Chicago Press.

Cowan, P. 1988. "In the Land of the Sick." *Village Voice*, May 17, 1988.

Dewey, J. 1988. *1938–1939: Experience and Education, Freedom and Culture, Theory of Valuation, and Essays*. Vol. 13 of *The Later Works, 1925–1954*. Edited by J. A. Boydston. Carbondale: Southern Illinois University Press.

Dubin, D. 1973. *Rapid Interpretation of EKGs*. 2nd ed. Tampa: Cover.

Fins, J. J. 1999. "Death and Dying in the 1990s: Intimations of Reality and Immortality." *Generations: Journal of the American Society on Aging* 23 (1): 81–86.

———. 2002. "A 38-Year-Old Man with a Secondary Leukemia Who Needs Setting of Goals of Care." In *Palliative and End-of-Life Pearls*, edited by J. E. Heffner and I. Byock, 174–76. Philadelphia: Hanley and Belfus.

———. 2006. *A Palliative Ethic of Care: Clinical Wisdom at Life's End*. Sudbury, MA: Jones and Bartlett.

———. 2007. "Ethics of Clinical Decision Making and Communication with Surrogates." In *Plum and Posner's Diagnosis of Stupor and Coma*, 4th ed., edited by J. B. Posner, C. B. Saper, N. D. Schiff, and F. Plum, 376–86. New York: Oxford University Press.

———. 2008. "Neuroethics and Disorders of Consciousness: A Pragmatic Approach to Neuro-Palliative Care." In *The Neurology of Consciousness: Cognitive Neuroscience and Neuropathology*, edited by S. Laureys and G. Tononi, 234–44. London: Academic Press.

———. 2014. "Private Decisions and Public Lessons." *CONSIDER: Magazine at the*

University of Michigan 30 (2). http://consideronline.org/assisted-suicide-is-it-ethical.

———. 2015. *Rights Come to Mind: Brain Injury, Ethics and the Struggle for Consciousness.* New York: Cambridge University Press.

———. 2017a. "My Time in Medicine." *Perspectives in Biology and Medicine* 60 (1): 19–32.

———. 2017b. "Towards a Pragmatic Neuroethics in Theory and Practice." In *The Debate About Neuroethics: Perspectives on the Field's Development, Focus, and Future,* edited by E. Racine and J. Aspler, 45–65. Berlin: Springer.

———. 2019a. "Disorders of Consciousness in Clinical Practice: Ethical, Legal and Policy Considerations." In *Plum and Posner's Diagnosis of Stupor and Coma,* 5th ed., edited by J. P. Posner, C. B. Saper, N. D. Schiff, and J. Claussen, 449–78. New York: Oxford University Press.

———. 2019b. "Disorders of Consciousness, Past, Present, and Future." *Cambridge Quarterly of Healthcare Ethics* 28 (4): 603–15.

———. 2019c. "When No One Notices: Disorders of Consciousness and the Chronic Vegetative State." *Hastings Center Report* 49 (4): 14–17.

———. 2020. "Saul Bellow's Coma: What Neuroscience Can Learn from the Humanities." *Journal of Head Trauma Rehabilitation* 35 (2): 160–62.

Fins, J. J., and J. L. Bernat. 2018. "Ethical, Palliative, and Policy Considerations in Disorders of Consciousness." *Neurology* 91 (10): 471–75. Simultaneously published in *Archives of Physical Medicine and Rehabilitation* 2018; 99 (9): 1927–31.

Fins, J. J., and M. G. Master. 2017. "Disorders of Consciousness and Neuro-Palliative Care: Towards an Expanded Scope of Practice for the Field." In *Oxford Handbook of Ethics at the End of Life,* edited by S. J. Youngner and R. Arnold, 154–69. New York: Oxford University Press.

Fins, J. J., F. G. Miller, C. A. Acres, M. D. Bacchetta, L. L. Huzzard, and B. D. Rapkin. 1999. "End-of-Life Decision-Making in the Hospital: Current Practices and Future Prospects." *Journal of Pain and Symptom Management* 17 (1): 6–15.

Fins, J. J., and M. B. Morrissey. 2018. "Reflections on 'Aid and Dying' and the Paradox of 'Achieving Death': Avoiding the Confluence of Language and Ideology at Life's End." *New York State Bar Association Health Law Journal* 23 (1): 59–65.

Fins, J. J., and F. Plum. 2004. "Neurological Diagnosis Is More than a State of Mind: Diagnostic Clarity and Impaired Consciousness." *Archives of Neurology* 61 (9): 1354–55.

Fins, J. J., and B. R. Pohl. 2015. "Neuro-Palliative Care and Disorders of Consciousness." In *Oxford Textbook of Palliative Medicine,* 5th ed., edited by G. Hanks, N. I. Cherny, N. A. Christakis, M. Fallon, S. Kassa, and R. K. Portenoy, 285–91. Oxford: Oxford University Press.

Fins, J. J., and N. D. Schiff. 2017. "Differences That Make a Difference in Disorders of Consciousness." *American Journal of Bioethics-Neuroethics* 8 (3): 131–34.

Giacino, J. T., D. I. Katz, N. D. Schiff, J. Whyte, E. J. Ashman, S. Ashwal, R. Barbano, F. M. Hammond, S. Laureys, G. S. F. Ling, R. Nakase-Richardson, R. T. Seel, S. Yablon, T. S. D. Getchius, G. S. Gronseth, and M. J. Armstrong. 2018a. "Comprehensive Systematic Review Update Summary: Disorders of Consciousness: Report of the Guideline Development, Dissemination, and Implementation Subcommittee of the American Academy of Neurology; the American Congress of Rehabilitation Medicine; and the National Institute on Disability, Independent Living, and Rehabilitation Research." *Neurology* 91 (10): 461–70. Simultaneously published in *Archives of Physical Medicine and Rehabilitation* 2018; 99 (9): 1710–19.

———. 2018b. "Practice Guideline Update Recommendations Summary: Disorders of Consciousness: Report of the Guideline Development, Dissemination, and Implementation Subcommittee of the American Academy of Neurology;

the American Congress of Rehabilitation Medicine; and the National Institute on Disability, Independent Living, and Rehabilitation Research. *Neurology* 91 (10): 450–60. Simultaneously published in *Archives of Physical Medicine and Rehabilitation* 2018; 99 (9): 1699–709.

Jennett, B., and F. Plum. 1972. "Persistent Vegetative State After Brain Damage: A Syndrome in Search of a Name." *Lancet* 1 (7753): 734–37.

Kierkegaard, S. 2003. *The Soul of Kierkegaard: Selections from His Journals.* Edited by A. Dru. Mineola, NY: Dover.

McGlinchey, L., ed. 2004. *Transforming the Culture of Dying: The Project on Death in America October 1994 to December 2003.* New York: Open Society Institute.

Morrison, R. S., M. D. Aldridge, J. Block, L. Chiu, C. Maroney, C. A. Morrison, and D. E. Meier. 2018. "The National Palliative Care Research Center: Ten Years of Promoting and Developing Research in Palliative Care." *Journal of Palliative Medicine* 21 (11): 1548–57.

Multi-Society Task Force on PVS. 1994a. "Medical Aspects of the Persistent Vegetative State (1)." *New England Journal of Medicine* 330 (21): 1499–508.

———. 1994b. "Medical Aspects of the Persistent Vegetative State (2)." *New England Journal of Medicine* 330 (22): 1572–79.

National Quality Forum. 2006. *A National Framework and Preferred Practices for Palliative and Hospice Care Quality: A Consensus Report.* Washington, DC: National Quality Forum.

Smith, J. E. 1969. "Time, Times and the 'Right Time': 'Chronos' and 'Kairos.'" *Monist* 53 (1): 1–13.

———. 2002. "Time and Qualitative Time." In *Rhetoric and Kairos: Essays in History, Theory, and Praxis,* edited by P. Sipiora and J. S. Baumlin, 46–57. Albany: State University of New York Press.

Swensen, S. J., G. S. Meyer, E. C. Nelson, G. C. Hunt Jr., D. B. Pryor, J. I. Weissberg, G. S. Kaplan, J. Daley, G. R. Yates, M. R. Chassin, B. C. James, and D. M. Berwick. 2010. "Cottage Industry to Postindustrial Care—The Revolution in Health Care Delivery." *New England Journal of Medicine* 362 (5): e12.

Turgeon, A. F., F. Lauzier, J.-F. Simard, D. C. Scales, K. E. A. Burns, L. Moore, D. A. Zygun, F. Bernard, M. O. Meade, T. C. Dung, M. Ratnapalan, S. Todd, J. Harlock, D. A. Fergusson, and Canadian Critical Care Trials Group. 2011. "Mortality Associated with Withdrawal of Life-Sustaining Therapy for Patients with Severe Traumatic Brain Injury: A Canadian Multicentre Cohort Study." *Canadian Medical Association Journal* 183 (14): 1581–88.

Wijdicks, E. F. M., and A. A. Rabinstein. 2007. "The Family Conference: End-of-Life Guidelines at Work for Comatose Patients." *Neurology* 68 (14): 1092–94.

Williams, T. 1966. *The Last of My Solid Gold Watches.* In *27 Wagons Full of Cotton and Other One-Act Plays,* 75–88. New York: New Directions Books.

———. 1999. *The Glass Menagerie.* New York: New Directions Books.

CHAPTER 6

Teaching Clinicians to Read

*How Narrative Medicine Prepares
Clinicians for Palliative Care*

Kathryn B. Kirkland

Patient narratives of illness and suffering can be disordered, incomplete, and difficult to make sense of. Clinicians are called upon to help patients order, complete, and make meaning of these stories but are not always well prepared to do so. Medical school and clinical training programs tend to teach information and knowledge currently believed to be true (but which is ultimately determined to be wrong about 50 percent of the time).[1] Curricula focus on pathophysiology, disease, certain types of evidence (e.g., randomized controlled trials), and outcomes more than patients' experiences of illness. Methods of teaching and of testing, and the emphasis on standardized licensing exams as measures of competence and ultimately mastery of material, tend to promote reductive, black-and-white thinking and the sense that there are right and wrong answers to all important questions. In medical schools and residency programs, communication training often emphasizes what to *say to* patients, with much less focus, if any, on how to *listen for* the concerns, values, and experiences of patients.

If "every system is perfectly designed to get the results that it gets,"[2] it should not be a surprise that we end up with clinicians who are trying to match patients with diagnostic categories, as quickly as possible, who often miss the subtleties of patient stories and fail to recognize the emotional responses to illness that their patients experience. In the case of palliative care, trainees often arrive to begin fellowship training unprepared to receive the stories of illness and suffering with which they are quickly confronted. Without training, they unconsciously substitute their own perspectives, what *they* would do or feel or how *they* would respond, for the patient's actual experience or reaction to the illness. For example, a new fellow might say, "I don't know what's wrong with this patient. She's not reacting to the news of metastatic cancer the way I would." Or, "How can he want to go through more surgery? I wouldn't!" Or, in response to a family decision, "It's terrible that they are putting her through all this!"

To become effective and empathic palliative care clinicians, it will be crucial for these fellows to learn or relearn a different set of responses: to be curious about perspectives and experiences other than their own; to pause in the face of tension, or ambiguity, or even suspense; to generate (and then be prepared to modify or discard) hypotheses and hunches.

How might we prepare these new clinicians to respond to the varied stories of illness, the range of emotional responses that we know our patients will experience? One way is by teaching them to read.

Reading exposes people to both familiar and unfamiliar worlds and offers opportunities to see problems and situations through different eyes. When we read, we meet characters who are like and unlike us, whom we like and don't like; we watch their responses to their own lives and watch the consequences of their choices play out. The more broadly clinicians read, the more their horizons of understanding and capacity to imagine a range of human experiences expand. This kind of exposure is what gives clinicians with a background in the humanities an advantage over those with a background only in science when they encounter a patient's story of illness.

But there is more to the case for teaching clinicians how to be better readers. Reading requires a set of skills that are directly transferable to the clinical setting. Practicing being a "mindful" reader, reading with self-awareness, openness, and humility, helps develop mindful listeners, clinicians who use these skills to deeply hear individual stories of illness and to provide person-centered, rather than simply disease-focused, care.

Thirty years ago, Rita Charon pointed out the parallels between patients and writers, doctors and readers.[3] She was an early advocate for teaching clinicians how to read closely, not just for content, but for form: language, metaphor, imagery, pace and tempo, mood, genre.[4] Charon's case was that learning to read enhanced clinicians' ability to receive, interpret, augment, and retell the stories of illness. In turn, she argued, this careful listening allows the development of affiliation between clinician and patient, and the development of relationships of mutual trust that are linked to better outcomes and experiences for patients.[5]

NARRATIVE PRACTICE AS SIMULATION LAB

In bygone times, clinical training of doctors often consisted of "See one, do one, teach one," an approach that perhaps valued experiential learning over patient safety. Nowadays, students and residents have the opportunity to practice skills, especially procedures that might present risks for patients, in simulation labs, on plastic dummies, before they are allowed to treat patients. While the risks of placing a central vascular catheter might be more obvious, unskilled communicators can also inflict harm, particularly when news is bad or decisions heart-wrenching. Fortunately, communication skills can also be learned and practiced safely using simulation training. Several components of the communication curriculum of our fellowship training program in hospice and palliative medicine take place in an actual simulation lab at Dartmouth-Hitchcock, where trainees practice serious illness conversations such as breaking bad news and dealing with emotional responses like anger, denial, and hopelessness, using standardized patients.[6]

An additional core component of communication training for our fellows, which has also been part of the curriculum for internal medicine and surgical residents, is in a different kind of "simulation lab," where we practice the narrative skills of close reading and writing, using poems, short fiction, paintings, or photographs as our texts. A typical narrative medicine session is one hour long and occurs during the workday. For the palliative care fellows, the sessions are part of their weekly "academic half-days," occurring approximately twice a month. Sessions with residents typically occur during lunchtime conference time. No prework or afterwork is expected. During each session a group of six to twenty people gathers around a table in a conference room. The sessions are structured using the framework long used and taught by the Columbia Narrative Medicine Program.[7] Each session revolves around a text short enough to be managed in a limited amount of time. The steps involve first reading the text closely as a group, paying attention not just to the story it tells, but to its form—language, images, mood, elements of time and movement.[8] After reading the poem in this way, the facilitator provides a writing prompt that is derived in some way from the text and designed to facilitate "free writing" about whatever comes to mind. Participants are asked to write for five to six minutes in response to this prompt. Afterward they are invited to share their writing with the group by reading it aloud. The group is instructed to listen as "close readers," not just for the content of their peers' writing but for elements of its form.

As structured, these sessions offer the opportunity for participants to practice a number of what can be considered narrative competencies, including those involved in reading (such as attention, curiosity, openness, patience, perspective-taking, humility, tolerance for ambiguity) and writing (accessing "the unthought known" of the unconscious mind).[9] In addition, by sharing their writing with peers, they practice vulnerability and build a community of practice.

WHAT HAPPENS WHEN WE READ?

Almost by chance, I have developed a variation in teaching methodology that has led to greater engagement of participants and deeper analysis of the texts. During an invited presentation about narrative medicine at Medicine Grand Rounds at Dartmouth, I facilitated a close reading of the first few lines of Jane Kenyon's poem "Coats,"[10] taking the audience through the lines one at a time. By slowing down the process, I created a space for more people to engage with the words, and we had a lively discussion during which many members of an audience of usually passive recipients shared widely differing perspectives on each line. A choice I had made for a formal presentation in order to limit the amount of time I spent demonstrating what close reading is led to my recognition of a potentially powerful new tool for my work with trainees, who often seem overwhelmed when asked to approach a poem in one huge chunk.

Since then, I've been experimenting with line-by-line close reading of poetry in my work with residents and fellows, curious about whether and how it might engage them more fully. In the process, I have learned much more about what happens when we read, and why it is so relevant to how we connect with patients to provide the best clinical care possible. Let's go now to the "narrative simulation lab" and watch as a group of residents reads and responds to a poem.

READING "COATS"

Twenty of us sit around a U-shaped conference room table. Pizza boxes are stacked on a table against the wall along with mostly empty bottles of soda. It's late spring, but warm weather has only just arrived; these trainees are close to the end of their year and eager for the transition ahead. The room hums with conversation as I hand out copies of the poem. The page is folded so that only the title is revealed, and as I pass them out I tell them not to unfold the papers. They gradually grow quiet, and I ask one of them to read the title out loud. "Coats," says the young man who volunteers. I ask them to close their eyes and see if an image comes to mind and then ask them to share those images. Around the table they tell what appeared in their mind's eye: for many of them it was a white coat, but others saw coats in a pile, discarded for the season, animal coats, coats of arms, coats of armor. We wonder aloud about whether the subject of the poem will turn out to be related to the images they saw.

Then we fold our papers down to reveal the first line of the poem, and another participant reads the title with the first line:

Coats

I saw him leaving the hospital

"What do you see now?" I ask. A number of them speak at once: "A resident leaving the hospital," one of them says. "Watching a patient leave the hospital," says another. "I'm imagining a patient watching from his window as people come and go, feeling jealous," says a third. "I have a sense of guilt," says the person next to her. I ask where these images are in the poem, pointing out that we are responding to just six words. It begins to dawn on them that these images are coming not from the poem itself, which is acting as a stimulus, but from their own experiences of seeing people leave a hospital. One of them points out that we are seeing this familiar scene through the eyes of a narrator, the "I" who opens the poem.

I point out that there is no punctuation ending the first line, and we talk about the effect of leaving a sentence incomplete like this. They see that it creates anticipation; for some it even creates a sense of dread about what might be coming. I give the group the technical name for this narrative technique—enjambment—and validate their feelings of suspense. We talk about the setting of the poem, how different its mood would be if it were a grocery store, a library, a school, and not a hospital. We speculate about what comes next.

I ask them to fold the paper to show one more line, and someone reads us from the title through the second line.

Coats

I saw him leaving the hospital
with a woman's coat over his arm.

Now, with completion of the first sentence, we have met three characters and have the beginning of a plot. "How do we know it is a woman's coat?" I ask. A vigorous discussion ensues, with various residents offering that the question can be answered by looking at which side the zipper is on, or suggesting that the color and pattern of the coat made it identifiable as a woman's. The group begins to hypothesize about the observer's perspective. They put themselves in his or her place: "I am walking in, and he is walking out," one says. Another sees the man leaving the hospital from a window, looking down from above. Another sits in a car outside the hospital waiting for someone else, watching people come and go. We notice how the narrator uses the pronoun "him," and not "a man," and argue about whether they know each other.

I ask them about the plot. "Is this a happy or a sad story?" One person spontaneously shares a story of someone who recently died in the intensive care unit, how he watched as the family left carrying her things. Another counters with a happy story, of someone having a baby. Leaving the question of mood unresolved, we turn to the third line of the poem, which the next resident reads aloud.

Coats

I saw him leaving the hospital
with a woman's coat over his arm.
Clearly she would not need it.

There is an immediate clamor of reactions to this line. "She totally died," says one resident. Others nod. "No—he left her there," says another, and a third, "No, the woman just said 'I don't need my coat.'" "Maybe it's summertime," says yet another, hopefully. We talk about the effect of the word "clearly." They see it as confidence, certainty. One of them shares his curiosity about the reliability of the person telling this story: "Can we trust him? How does he know?" A lot hinges on these questions. How we interpret the story depends on who is seeing, who is telling, and his or her claim to authority.

We move on and another resident reads us through line 4:

Coats

I saw him leaving the hospital
with a woman's coat over his arm.
Clearly she would not need it.
The sunglasses he wore could not

Whereas they all missed the enjambment on the first line, none of them misses it this time. In fact, many express frustration at the way the story is left hanging in this moment. Figures 6.1 and 6.2 show the line-by-line notes of two residents. We can see their interactions with the text, their unfolding hypotheses, framed in more or less conditional language and with evidence of self-correction ("Close.") when the fifth line is revealed.

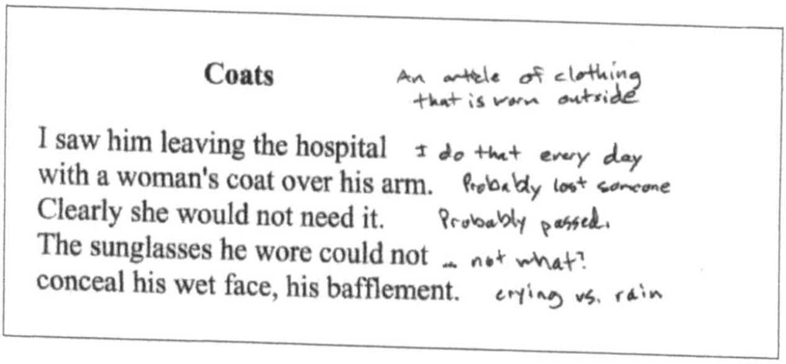

Coats   An article of clothing
                that is worn outside

I saw him leaving the hospital   I do that every day
with a woman's coat over his arm.   Probably lost someone
Clearly she would not need it.   Probably passed.
The sunglasses he wore could not ... not what?
conceal his wet face, his bafflement.   crying vs. rain

FIG. 6.1 One resident's line-by-line notes on the first stanza of "Coats."

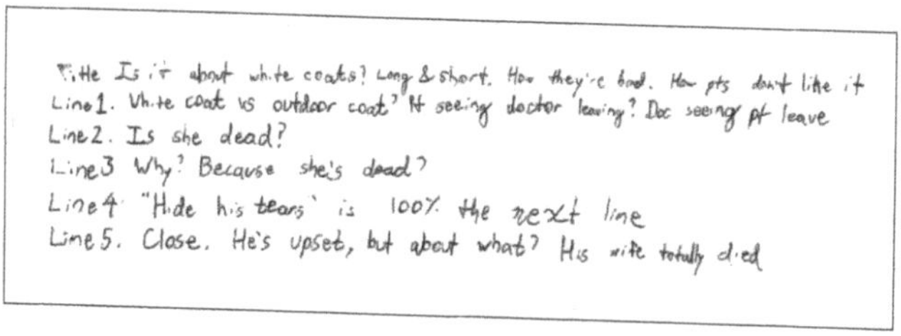

Title Is it about white coats? Long & short. How they're bad. How pts don't like it
Line 1. White coat is outdoor coat? It seeing doctor 'leaving'? Doc seeing pt leave
Line 2. Is she dead?
Line 3 Why? Because she's dead?
Line 4 "Hide his tears" is 100% the next line
Line 5. Close. He's upset, but about what? His wife totally died

FIG. 6.2 A second resident's line-by-line notes on the first stanza of "Coats."

After reading the first stanza line by line, we reveal the second stanza as a whole, in order to leave time for a short writing exercise. The poem in its entirety is as follows:

I saw him leaving the hospital
with a woman's coat over his arm.
Clearly she would not need it.
The sunglasses he wore could not
conceal his wet face, his bafflement.

As if in mockery the day was fair,
and the air mild for December. All the same
he had zipped his own coat and tied
the hood under his chin, preparing
for irremediable cold.[11]

Our discussion starts with the word "fair," and its multiple meanings. We notice the ways that the rhythms change, with multiple successive syllables competing for emphasis, making it challenging to read aloud. We end our discussion with the unambiguous words "irremediable cold." "Weather is always temporary, so this is metaphorical cold," one of them says. By this point, anyone who has been clinging to the possibility that this poem tells a happy story tends to let go of their hypothesis. In response to my question about the mood the poem creates, they offer one-word answers: isolated, grief, lonely, despair, loss.

Finally we go back to reconsider the title in light of the poem as a whole. Their thoughts turn metaphorical as they offer ideas about coats as protective coverings, ways of hiding or retreating from the world, and legacies (he is left with a coat to remind him of what he had).

Ideally, we have about fifteen minutes left to write and share our writing. The writing exercise is not to write *about* the poem but to write in its shadow, in response to a writing prompt. Although I've found that essentially any text can work as the subject of a close-reading exercise, there is a real art to creating good writing prompts. The role of a prompt is to stimulate creative, free, reflective writing. The most effective prompts borrow language from the text or, in the case of a visual prompt (artwork or a photograph), relate to something specific in its content. While it should be specific to the text, it works best if it is not overly narrow or prescriptive. The goal is to create a prompt to which a group of individuals with a wide range of experiences can respond. In this case, I ask the group to "write about something that will not be needed." The things they write about that will not be needed range from trips to India, to size 6 months baby clothes, to our bodies, to "my grandmother's treasures." Many but not all relate to death or loss; a few are humorous, many wistful or poignant. A minority address things that relate to medical practice or their day-to-day work.

READING AS TRANSACTION

Narrative theory, particularly reader-writer theory, helps illuminate what happens when residents engage, line-by-line, with a poem and provides insight into why narrative exercises might be good practice for clinical care. In her book *The Reader, the Text, the Poem: The Transactional Theory of the Literary Work*,[12] Louise Rosenblatt describes what happens when she gives her literature students a four-line poem, "It Bids Pretty Fair," by Robert Frost, and asks them to write down their thinking as they read and make sense of the lines. Her exercise reveals thought processes quite similar to those I have seen as groups of doctors read poetry one line at a time. Confronted with a new text, these students, just like the group of residents reading "Coats," actively engaged with it, drawing on their own experiences of life and literature to try to make meaning out of the words. Like the interns, they moved back and forth among the lines, understanding the first line differently after reading the fourth. They developed hypotheses as they read, then subjected them to reassessment as the lines unfolded.

Rosenblatt proposes that a "poem" emerges only when a reader interacts with a text, and I would submit that in a parallel way, a narrative of illness emerges only when a "reader-clinician" interacts with a patient story or text. Rosenblatt argues that the text serves both as a stimulus, activating the reader's past experiences and imagination, and as a blueprint, serving to regulate the selection, rejection, and ordering of which experiences are relevant. She points out the need for rigor in this process of "creating" a narrative, insisting that the reader, who necessarily brings all his past experiences and all the literature he has read before to each new encounter with a text, must be faithful to the text. This faithfulness extends not just to the content of the text, according to Rosenblatt, but to its particular order and form.

A clinician must be no less rigorous in constructing meaning, attending not just to the content of her patient's story, its plot and characters, but also to its chronology, its pace, its images, its silences. As a literature student brings his experiences of reading and of life to an encounter with a text, a clinician brings to each patient story an array of her own medical narratives of clinical experience, of pathophysiology and of evidence, using them to generate and test hypotheses that impart meaning to the narratives of illness. Careful to keep the text at the center, a reader must subject his hypotheses to self-critique and self-correction. Similarly, a clinician's obligation is to ensure that her evolving hypotheses remain true to the story told by her patient. The clinician could be said to have the advantage of an ongoing relationship with the author of the text with which she works; this comes also with the added complexity of reading a story that may still be unfolding, and the telling of which—and the meaning of which—may change in real time.

A second concept Rosenblatt introduces in her book[13] seems equally relevant to the training of clinicians. Rosenblatt describes two kinds of reading processes, appropriate for different purposes. Efferent reading is reading for information; its goal is the "residue," or the points to be taken away. Rosenblatt's example for efferent reading is reading the instructions for a fire extinguisher: the purpose is to gain the information needed to use the device. Speed and efficiency are of high value in this case. Aesthetic reading, on the other hand, is reading with a focus on the experience of reading itself, what happens between the reader and the text that yields meaning, feelings, deeper understanding. Clinicians are traditionally trained to be efferent readers, reading efficiently to derive information, to determine the right answer, to learn how to perform a task. Efferent reading is an inarguably critical clinical competency. I would propose that learning to read aesthetically is equally critical for clinicians, who need to engage with the stories of illness experience in order to make meaning and care for the whole person suffering from the disease.

NARRATIVE MEDICINE FOR PALLIATIVE MEDICINE

The processes literature students and medical trainees use when they encounter literary texts are remarkably similar and reflect the possibility that in every encounter between human and story, it is only through the interaction of the two that meaning is co-created. If this is true, the use of narrative medicine sessions as a simulation lab for developing narrative skills that can be used in clinical encounters makes sense. Beyond the development of efferent and aesthetic reading skills, the participation with peers in activities that involve developing hypotheses about the meaning of a text brings clinical trainees face-to-face with the way that their own experiences, values, and beliefs color their interpretations of texts. Over time, as they confront conflicts between their own and others' interpretations of texts, conflicts that cannot be resolved into right and wrong answers, they develop a capacity to seek out and be curious about different perspectives and to tolerate ambiguity and uncertainty.

The practice of palliative care requires all of these competencies. The integration of narrative exercises as a regular part of the fellowship curriculum helps prepare fellows to create space for the sometimes chaotic and unexpected stories of individual patients with serious illness and to engage with them as open-minded readers. Their narrative skills are also evident in the ways they engage with the narratives of others on our interprofessional team and on the services with whom we share patients, creating the conditions for sustainable, empathic, and even joyful work.

NOTES

1. Attributed to David Sackett.
2. IHI Multimedia Team 2015.
3. Charon 1989.
4. Charon 2006; Charon, Hermann, and Devlin 2016.
5. Charon 2006.
6. Vergo et al. 2017.
7. Charon 2006; Charon, Hermann, and Devlin 2016.
8. Charon, Hermann, and Devlin 2016.
9. Bollas 1987.
10. Jane Kenyon, "Coats," from *Collected Poems*. Copyright © 2005 by The Estate of Jane Kenyon. Reprinted with the permission of The Permissions Company, LLC on behalf of Graywolf Press, graywolfpress.org.
11. Kenyon 1993.
12. Rosenblatt 1978.
13. Ibid.

WORKS CITED

Bollas, C. 1987. *The Shadow of the Object: Psychoanalysis of the Unthought Known.* London: Free Association Books.

Charon, R. 1989. "Doctor-Patient/Reader-Writer: Learning to Find the Text." *Soundings* 72 (1): 137–52.

———. 2006. *Narrative Medicine: Honoring the Stories of Illness.* Oxford: Oxford University Press.

Charon, R., N. Hermann, and M. J. Devlin. 2016. "Close Reading and Creative Writing in Clinical Education: Teaching Attention, Representation, and Affiliation." *Academic Medicine* 91 (3): 345–50.

IHI Multimedia Team. "Like Magic? ('Every System Is Perfectly Designed...')." *Institute for Healthcare Improvement* (blog), August 21, 2015. http://www.ihi

.org/communities/blogs/origin-of
-every-system-is-perfectly-designed
-quote.

Kenyon, J. 1993. "Coats." In *Constance*.
Minneapolis: Graywolf Press.

Rosenblatt, L. 1978. *The Reader, the Text, the
Poem: The Transactional Theory of the
Literary Work*. Carbondale: Southern
Illinois University Press.

Vergo, M. T., S. Sachs, M. A. MacMartin, K. B.
Kirkland, A. M. Cullinan, and L. A.
Stephens. 2017. "Acceptability and
Impact of a Required Palliative Care
Rotation with Prerotation and
Postrotation Observed Structured
Clinical Experience During Internal
Medicine Residency Training on
Primary Palliative Communication
Skills." *Journal of Palliative Medicine* 20
(5): 542–47.

CHAPTER 7

Sophocles, Hospice, and the Call of the Body

Joseph Calandrino

AN INVITATION

"This is my body."
"Do not kill me."
"Do not euthanize me."
"I am still here."
"Don't be frightened, it's still me."
"This is the same me you know."
"This is what I've become."
"This is what happened to me."
"I am the same person now that I was then."
"Hold, enough—do not pretend to give me more life."
"See me."
"Recognize me."

Suffering and dying bodies speak. They call out to us, demanding that we see them, listen to them, recognize them.

The voice of the suffering body has no specific language; rather, the voice speaks a wordless yet intelligible *body* language. With neither syntax nor lexicon, the charged language of *the body*, voiced in tones of human suffering and plaintive personhood, "says" many things at once. The voice of the suffering body calls to every human person who comes near.

Time might occasionally heal a wound or two, but time cannot blunt the edge of human suffering or its pointed call voiced to be heard and recognized. This is a call whose appeal has been heard from time immemorial; certainly, the ancients knew it. Nearly two and half millennia separate us today, for example, from the Greek playwright Sophocles. Perhaps his greatest play, *Philoctetes*, asks the same questions of human suffering, the human body, and human personhood we continue to ask today, especially as we care for those who suffer from life-threatening illness, for those who are dying.

What has Greek tragedy to do with hospice care? This essay explores suffering and personhood in *Philoctetes* and traces the discoveries made there—by the playwright, his characters, and his audience—into the experience of several patients who spent their last weeks on our hospice and palliative care unit. We will see the human person, exposed and wounded, giving voice to a relentless call seeking a healing response through the recognition of the wholeness of the human person. It is a voice Sophocles heard long ago on the Aegean; it is one we still hear today wherever humans suffer.

EXILE AND EMPATHY IN THE ANCIENT WORLD

Sophocles's tragedy *Philoctetes* illuminates the experience of the suffering human and the way in which the suffering body of another calls out to us and voices itself as a unique person. The tragedian pits human suffering in exile against a cultural setting conflicted in the face of such suffering. The characters and their situations grip us today as powerfully as they did for the audience in ancient Athens. Indeed, *Philoctetes* enjoys a place not only in the canon of Western literature but also in the canon of the literature of medical ethics, medical humanities, and the training of medical students.[1]

The tragedy presents the effort to enlist Philoctetes in the Trojan War after his abandonment on the desert island of Lemnos by Odysseus, one of the same characters now seeking to bring him to Troy. Odysseus, along with Agamemnon and Menelaus, had exiled Philoctetes because of a festering wound he received from a snakebite when he carelessly stepped on sacred ground on the island of Chryse. Philoctetes's relentless screams of pain and the oozing wound itself compelled the Greeks to abandon him, even at the expense of Philoctetes's skills. Odysseus explains to Neoptolemus, the son of Achilles:

> *His foot*
> *diseased and eaten away with running ulcers.*
>
> . . . .
>
> *We had no peace with him: at the holy festivals,*
> *we dared not touch the wine and meat; he screamed*
> *and groaned so, and those terrible cries of his*
> *brought ill luck on our celebrations; all*
> *the camp was haunted by him. (5–10)²*

Upon learning that the war will be lost without the bow of Heracles, which is in Philoctetes's possession, the Greeks plot to bring Philoctetes and the bow to Troy by any means possible; failing that, they will at least steal Heracles's bow. They enlist the young Neoptolemus in their treachery, and he goes along with the plan—at least initially.

THE ADVENT OF EMPATHY

Odysseus's unflattering appearance here in *Philoctetes*—he is not Homer's driven hero struggling to return to home and hearth—stands for subterfuge, for a "by hook or by crook" expediency, advancing the imperatives of his culture. Both Odysseus and Neoptolemus respond to Philoctetes's plight, yet only the latter responds to the suffering of his body as it defines both body and personhood. Neoptolemus and Odysseus, in fact, receive Philoctetes and his suffering differently. Odysseus remains closed off, encountering the other as more of the same, business as usual. Neoptolemus opens himself to the closeness of the other—suffering and festering Philoctetes—and encounters difference instead. In contrast to Odysseus, Achilles's young son Neoptolemus offers a consolation that conflicts with the needs of Odysseus's world.

The confines of Odysseus's culture, whose edges sharpen in the throes of war, and his own senses limit the manner and content of the appearance of Philoctetes's suffering. Odysseus already knows what he will experience before he experiences it; irresistible cultural imperatives prescribe the parameters of the experience for him, and he does not violate them. He can neither tolerate nor understand—let alone empathize with—the deep emotions of pain and suffering.

However, Neoptolemus permits his experience to take shape apart from the cultural paradigm he ostensibly shares with Odysseus. He allows Philoctetes's "burden" to appear in its true abundance, a "burden" that simply overwhelms Odysseus's worldview. For Neoptolemus, Philoctetes's body, his stinking wound and grating howls, speak on their own terms: he experiences them as they present themselves in their absolute starkness, which inflicts a wound upon his conscience, a wound of inner conflict.

Neoptolemus experiences Philoctetes's "terrible burden of [his] sickness" (753) on its own terms, and this experience begins a process of transformation. He witnesses the wound and its "blood . . . trickling, dripping murderously," accompanied by agonizing screams (783). Faced with growing reluctance to participate in the plan to trick Philoctetes, Neoptolemus finds both a strange sympathy and empathy. He can now say to Philoctetes, "I have been in pain for you; I have been / in sorrow for your pain" (805–6). Neoptolemus's remarkable distinction between an empathetic being "in pain" and a sympathetic "sorrow for" pain shapes the younger man's experience of this other person before him. This experience takes Neoptolemus beyond a mere response to "human suffering," and he encounters more than a *concept* of misery. He receives and responds to the very presence of human tissue spewing forth its guts.[3] Because he does not limit his own response to the merely visceral, more than the visceral can appear—human personhood can now appear from the very substance of suffering.

The character and utterances of Philoctetes are therefore only superficial. The experience of the oneness of the person comes instead from the depths of the body, from its own "deep spring" (784). The voice, blood, stench, moan— these expressions of the wounded body conspire to move Achilles's son to return to his better nature and to come clean with his new friend. The young man discovers compassion and true pity for Philoctetes (960–70), whom he recognizes in his wholeness of personhood: not simply a tool to win a war but a suffering human being. This ethical moment arises neither from a passing feeling nor a cognitive event but from the transformative power of this wounded body, whose voice claims Neoptolemus, as it grabs him and leads him to a change of heart and a change of course.

Philoctetes comes to realize that he will be going to Troy after all. Faced finally with the prospect of his departure from Lemnos, he gathers his thoughts and his belongings. The fascinating moment of searching for his comforting herbs and his misplaced arrows illustrates how a wound in and of itself directs action and character. The search makes practical sense: the herbs palliate the wound and arrows feed the bow. Neoptolemus invites him to take the items he most needs and loves.

> *A herb I have, the chief means to soothe my wound,*
> *to lull the pain to sleep.*
>
> . . . .
>
> *Any arrow*
> *I may have dropped and missed. For none of them*
> *must I leave.* (649–55)

Wound and person gel in these lines spoken to Neoptolemus, as the herbs and arrows underscore the oozing wound's power to dictate the action: "The sickness in me seeks to have you beside me" (675–76). Both characters enter the cave, where the wound and wounded appear graphically in excruciating sound and sight. Neoptolemus experiences the connection between body and wound, wound and person, and he distinguishes the body as a simple extension of personhood from a body vividly inhabited, a corpus vividly lived.

THE AGONY OF RELEASE

Philoctetes would measure his lifetime on Lemnos with each storied arrow he recovers, as he plucks each one from the wounded substance of the wilderness that sustained him. Each arrow becomes valediction and closure, a remedy for wounded pride and prideful wound. His emotional farewell to Lemnos, which had become for him sustenance and sympathetic companion in his loneliness, punctuates the healing of a wounded landscape that reflected his own pain for ten years:

> *Farewell, cave that shared my watches,*
> *nymphs of the meadow and the stream,*
> *the deep male growl of the sea-lashed headland*
> *where often, in my niche within the rock,*
> *my head was wet with fine spray,*

where many a time in answer to my crying
in the storm of my sorrow the Hermes mountain sent its echo! (1452–60)

The search and recovery of Philoctetes's arrows make plain to the characters and audience alike that he will fulfill his civic duty and find his rightful place of honor among the Greeks. The pressure builds within each protagonist until each recognizes the *injury* within himself and within each other. This shifting paradigm leads to transformation and righteous action—and finally to healing.

THE WOUND IN THE OTHER

Both Philoctetes and Neoptolemus recognize the wound in the other as a brokenness within each man crying out to be heard: a voice pointing to wounds not only of bodily tissue but also of conscience. Yet neither character is simply healed by healing the other. These are not wounded healers who through healing the other effect their own healing.+ Sophocles forecloses on that reading by putting the injuries themselves center stage, not the human will to heal. The two characters pledge to obey the voice of the body's suffering not merely in deference to divine command but in response to the givenness of the other's suffering. The action of the drama unfolds in the recognition of wounds that are not mere marks upon bodies but connect deeply and absolutely with the personhood within such wounds.

Neoptolemus acknowledges that his "terrible compassion" for Philoctetes did not begin in the wounded heel alone but already in the history he learns about his elder's plight, something he has felt for him "all the time" (968). Yet his transformation only occurs fully when that history is reunited with the body of the man. So, too, with Philoctetes, who hears the call of anguish from the younger man,

who knows nothing but to do what he was bidden
and now, you see, is suffering bitterly,
for his own faults. (1010–11)

The tragedy, then, presents actions of healing and of personal transformation in response to recognizing the wholeness of the human other—the transformational unfolding of the human body, the unraveling of its voice, and the uncompromising claim of its call to be heard, seen, and recognized.

Experiencing the wound and its voice, Neoptolemus does not merely "see and hear" but is himself seen and heard. He does not merely see his own brokenness, his own fractured body in the mode of a cracking conscience; he is *seized* by the call from the oozing heel. Because he has acknowledged this wound as marked in the lived body of a person, an event of transformation becomes possible. This transformation, begun already in Neoptolemus's experience of being "in pain" for Philoctetes and feeling "sorrow for" him, now moves him to break with subterfuge and treachery and instead to pursue the more honorable course.

By contrast, Odysseus, who mistrusts the body, sees only his own reflection in the wound, experiencing its putrefaction as a pollution in his world, a disruption in civil society, where festivities must not be bothered by stench and scream. By forcing the body into social convention, Odysseus shuts himself off from growth, knowledge, and feeling anything for another.

These contrasting receptions of the suffering and wounded body either free or restrict what gives itself in every line of the drama. For Odysseus, Philoctetes's personhood and the call voiced by his wound go unnoticed. Neoptolemus and Philoctetes, instead, face and confront each other; they hear the self that presents a demand through the fractures of the body: the voice that commands the recognition of a unique suffering human person.

EXILE IN OUR WORLD

Much of what goes on in Sophocles's play also occurs on the horizons of life and death as they appear, for example, on the hospice unit, where people receive the highly specialized care of life-threatening, personhood-threatening illness; where they live on the continuum of suffering, dying, and death. Such suffering occurs everywhere the human body is, transcending place and time. Though the ancient world seems remote, it remains a world both familiar and strange to us. The problem of the body did not escape it. In many ways, seriously ill patients today also live as if exiled by, for, and with their illness. They mark time with the rudiments of survival: bow, arrow, a photograph, a familiar pillow or blanket. The routines of care and thoughts of themselves in the past, present, and future become their only consolation. Patients live out many of the images and themes in *Philoctetes* every day. They navigate diseases that threaten to take them down the darkling abyss of total desolation and loss. All those who sit at the bedside—doctors, nurses, friends, and family—encounter the brokenness of the body. The body's call obligates them—should they care to listen.

Crystal: Marked in the Body

Crystal was a thirty-five-year-old woman who suffered and eventually died from AIDS. Anatomically, Crystal's body had both male and female features; yet she lived her body as a woman, which put her at great risk for contracting the illness that caused her suffering and death. She could no longer speak, but she announced her awareness of my presence by slowly opening one eye. She was emaciated, moribund, and powerful. Her gaze upon me put me on notice, but the voice stirring from within and beyond those languishing eyes commanded a special attention. This call, a call for a recognition of who she was, someone more and otherwise than this ravaged body that betrayed her at every moment—this call, unique to her, could come from her alone. This call emanated from this very singular self through this singular body. The word *this*, this ordinary word, has the power to direct, to point, to lead. I stood before not just any Crystal, but this Crystal, this body of hers, and this call directing me, pointing me to this person in this body. The uncanny property of *this* endowed Crystal's eyes with a gaze and voice that positioned me to see *her*, not as a dying body, wasting and sexually ambiguous, but in her radiance as a woman concluding her life, not as a mass of failing organs and bodily functions, but in the wholeness of her singular personhood.

In that moment, Crystal invited me to participate in her healing before she died. She located her very self beyond the failing of her organicity, beyond the disintegration of body systems, and within the manner she lived her body. Her life proved that gender is marked not in the anatomical body but in that body lived out in her world.

The "deep spring" of Crystal's lived body unmistakably identified the stakes in the experience of dying, and the experience on the part of others who witnessed that dying and death. This was the same "deep spring" from which Philoctetes's wound, person, and lived experience emerged to become visible to Achilles's son. I cannot hear a call or feel a gaze from another if I do not first experience the autonomous uniqueness of that other. Neoptolemus's uncanny experience of seeing and hearing, and being seen and heard, played out in the dramatic action in Crystal's end of life. Crystal's opening eye was both a window and a two-way mirror. Beyond her jaundiced eye was a human *self* calling over the din of dying tissue, trying to get itself heard, vying for recognition, vying to express a wholeness of personhood against the cacophony of disintegration, vying to be recognized and therefore healed. My response ratified the power of her call; only then could I recognize her from the deep spring, the source, of her suffering.

Maurice: The Dignity of Personhood

Maurice was on the hospice unit for about two weeks when his wife approached me and said, "We decided that Friday at 2PM would be a good time."

I responded, "Hello, good morning; would you tell me more about what you mean by that?"

"We're ready for the injection," she said.

Acknowledging that some new point had been reached, I said, "Oh, I see; has something changed?"

"Well, enough is enough already, and we're prepared," she said.

I nodded and asked, "Why don't we sit down in the family room, where you can help me understand what's been going on?"

The conversation that ensued entailed a request for death in the face of the profound loss of personal autonomy and dignity. Maurice received some of his care, his more intimate care, only with humiliation and existential suffering. His organic functions, of his bladder and bowel, were no longer under his control. They forced a confrontation with his will, his self, his lived body. So tied to his dignity was the ability to wash himself and perform the routine activities of hygiene that the loss of this ability was tantamount to a loss, not only of his dignity, but of personhood itself. His body, though shot through with a spreading tumor that weakened his bones and drained his strength, remained outwardly intact, untouched by the wasting associated with advanced cancer, but the nakedness and exposure of that body to the hospice staff became increasingly unbearable to him. His body assumed the posture of invisible gashes and a denuding of his personhood, and it called for an end of the body that matched the end of his suffering self.

The task before all of us—Maurice, his family, and the palliative care team—was to find a safe harbor for Maurice's dignity and wholeness of person that would allow him to receive care without devastating loss. We discussed the nonjudgmental and objective approach professional caregivers give to their patients, which as such would not threaten him with loss of modesty of the body and an underscoring of lost autonomy. We also discussed how Maurice might relocate the sources of autonomy and dignity elsewhere, away from the necessary hygienic care he required daily. The request for death dissolved in this dislocation and relocation. He stayed on the hospice unit many weeks, and he was able to find a wholeness of self by redefining what professional care, however intimate in nature, meant for him. By uncoupling the anguish of loss from the reception of personal care, Maurice placed the locus of meaning in his story—his personal narrative—*elsewhere*, and he and his family were able to work with the treatment team toward a healing prior to his death.

Maurice's body, splayed, displayed and vulnerable, provided the avenue by which his very self sought exit.[5] Now, at the end of his life, Maurice realigned his personhood with his body that was broken and dying. His personhood came at me most fully through this body, whose voice traveled the waves of pure organic body, the medium of a unique message from a unique person asserting itself, as Philoctetes, so long ago, had done. Both men, seemingly removed from each other by time, share the same moment of finding a way to move forward.

Vincent: A Wound Deeper than Skin and Bone

Vincent was a sixty-eight-year-old man admitted to the hospice unit for end-of-life care while suffering his two end-stage cancers: cancer of the prostate and lymphoma. His goal was to have his symptoms of pain and shortness of breath lessened, so that he could visit with family and friends. His disease was quite advanced, and not only did he suffer from the wasting of his body, that body itself began quite literally to break down: the skin on his back had fallen away; plainly visible were fascia, muscles, tendon, and bone. This denuding of his tissue, remarkably, caused him little pain; it was the care of what was left of his back that caused him to moan and sometimes writhe in pain, until his pain medication was adjusted to peak at the time of his wound care. The wound was cleaned and dressed periodically. Topical disinfectants and antibiotics quelled the stench of dead and dying tissue. He was positioned in his bed to offload pressure on the gigantic wound, but he preferred to spend some time reclining in bed, on his back.

One of the sticky issues here was how to palliate Vincent's gaping wound without covering over (to "cover" is the etymological heart of "palliation") what the wound *meant*. We needed to locate the importance of his wound in acts of palliation without relegating the wound to invisibility, negating it. To negate the wound would in some way be a negation of Vincent. As in *Philoctetes*, the connection between wound and person does not dissolve. The wound therefore required a certain kind of care, not merely a correct putting out of sight, to hide the wound, to exile it elsewhere.

Vincent could not see the large swath of disintegrated body that replaced what was once his back; he suffered his wound not as pain or as humiliation (for the intimate attention it commanded of his nurses) but as the reach of the pure threat that was consuming him—and that would eventually kill him. Part of him had gone missing. He would sometimes speak of "what's left of me" in terms of what remained of himself to visit with loved ones. "I don't want to scare anyone," he once commented. It was important to him, therefore, that he not look as sick as he was. He wanted to speak with people whom he did not want distracted by the disfigurement seeping into the very air that surrounded him, signaling his impending death. In this sense, Vincent enjoyed the clean, sterile dressings that covered what was ugly and frightening and the medications that lessened the smell of his wound, the reeking of dying that infiltrated his space.

The white lies of palliation are the most forgivable of sins. In themselves, they were not delusion or denial but a strategy that held death at bay, that allowed for the continuation of dying without the tremors of death. Vincent was coping without lying to himself. Each day he bared his back to care, he opened himself to be seen, truly seen. Wound care suppressed nothing but instead released the power of the wound to reveal the middle ground between the body lived and the body proper, which extends into the world as the entry point of all our human and personal acts. Vincent's body, exploded and expanded in his wound, presented for care against the linens of his bed, told a truth far greater than any lie that might be in play.

My experience of Vincent's suffering cannot be identical with his suffering as lived by him; no sympathy or empathy can penetrate the lived body of the other. As Neoptolemus learned so long ago, sympathy and empathy are not qualities I bring to the encounter with another, but instead arise de novo each time I am directed, positioned by a call. Indeed, this call puts into question more than sympathy or empathy. My presence, directed by this call from his body spread out on his bed, my very self now positioned to be Vincent's witness, receives his personhood, once hidden by the brokenness of his body. This is the selfsame obligation Neoptolemus felt as Philoctetes's wound and suffering accused him, leading to his witnessing and recognizing the call of his friend's personhood. The voice calls me into question, accuses me and obligates me to recognize Vincent, this Vincent whose story I have heard, whom I have treated. Like Neoptolemus before Philoctetes's wound and howls of suffering, I find myself in the perfect position to see better, to see more, to recognize this living personhood before me. This pointing-me-toward and pointing-toward-me charges me with an invitation: a hospitality asking for hospitality.

This recognition, called for and effected by the call of his broken and exposed organicity, brings both Vincent and me into a moment of welcome, a moment of healing. In the sympathy and empathy originating from Vincent's call, I recognize Vincent among the ruins of body and time, and, in the event of his call, he is in turn recognized, restored to his just place. His person is again incarnated; his spread, sprawled body recedes as his lived body resurfaces from the abyss of threat. He is healed as he moves toward death: the paradox of healing in dying.

AN INVITATION TO SUFFERING AND PALLIATION

The protagonists in Sophocles's tragedy, as well as Crystal, Maurice, and Vincent, offer a call that emanates from their very personhoods. The experience of the wounds and sounds of suffering challenges our acceptance of illness (and dying) in both the ancient world and our own. The past illuminates the present; the present reads the past. Bodies read bodies across time. The exposed and vulnerable body points to something beyond it, putting into experience that body's forceful gaze upon me. In this experience of hearing and being heard, of seeing and being seen, the body connects me to the singular personhood whose voice comes from this disintegrating body as the force of a call. The breaking and brokenness of the suffering body deliver human personhood, inseparable from its organic, material body, and it appears in an assertion of a particular self. This call speaks both through and from this body under threat, which positions me to see and hear. I am myself seen and heard, called to task, called to recognize the uniqueness of the other person.

The suffering human body seeks healing, not restoration, especially in the face of a disease that is lethal. Though Sophocles's Philoctetes will be cured of his wound and returned to a heroic life that will pass into myth, the heroism of hospice patients rests in a different order. Such heroes will pass into the memory of family, friends, and physicians (indeed, all the professional caregivers who work closely with patients on the hospice unit). Their heroism resides in the assertion of the wholeness of personhood calling from the dying body. The recognition of this heroic assertion has no agenda apart from its assuming the shape of a response to the call. The claim on me positions me to recognize a person.

This recognition follows not from anything I initiate, but from the profound humanity of the other person. The uncanny calling voice of a suffering human person positions me to see, to hear, to recognize this person before me, who calls uncompromisingly. My presence can take the form of empathy—the experience of the pain of another. My presence can take the form, too, of sympathy—compassion for the pain of another. My presence is what counts. My honest, earnest, attentive presence.

The physician must acknowledge the uniqueness of the other person and resist the desire to master, to exert control over the biological basis of the living body as composed of parts and processes. Such attempts are futile anyway, as the body on the hospice unit thwarts manipulations of the physiologies and chemistries that work in the *curing* approaches usually deployed by medicine. Indeed, on the hospice unit, all that is left is *caring*. And caring is hearing and seeing; the hearing and seeing that Sophocles presented at Athens to his world.

Neither the deserted landscape of Lemnos, the site of Philoctetes's exile, nor the hospice unit—the spaces where the voice of the body echoes—gives the body its voice. Rather, *the body*, whose voice creates such spaces, defines the very limits of these spaces. The body forges its own reason for being, generating the unconditional force of its call. I must pass through this suffering of the material body spread out, broken, and yearning, in order to hear its unique call, which discloses a personhood that demands a response. This personhood makes a claim on me and prompts me to experience its fullness. The call of the wounded body places me on notice and marks the locus where my own gaze is transfixed by the gaze of another.

This call, this voice, is the call and voice of every human person. We all suffer death; we all die calling.

NOTES

1. One need look no further than, for example, Malpas and Lickiss 2012, but countless volumes abound.

2. Sophocles 1968. Line numbers will be given in parentheses in the body of the text.

3. The concept of "givenness," in this essay dubbed "presence," pertains to the work of Marion, especially as articulated in his *Being Given: Toward a Phenomenology of Givenness* (2002). The presence of the body is given in such a way as to come purely from itself, of itself, and it shows itself apart from any imprint from its receiver or reception.

4. For an interesting take on such a phenomenon, see Kearney 2016, 15–26. Sophocles's characters are indeed wounded, and they do "heal," but the relationship between wounds and healing differs sharply from that relation in Kearney's treatment. The piece contains a fascinating discussion of the Hippocratic and Asclepian modes of healing.

5. See Falque's analytic of the splayed, expanded body in his descriptions of experiences on a hospice unit in his essay "Ethics of the Spread Body" (2019). See also his *Ethique du corps epandu* (2018).

WORKS CITED

Falque, E. 2018. *Ethique du corps epandu*. Paris: Cerf.

———. 2019. "Ethics of the Spread Body." In *Somatic Desire: Rethinking Corporeality in Contemporary Thought*, edited by S. Horton, S. Mendelsohn, C. Rojewicz, and R. Kearney, 91–116. Lanham, MD: Lexington Press.

Kearney, R. 2016. "Wounded Healers." *Japan Mission Journal* 70 (1): 15–26.

Malpas, J., and N. Lickiss, eds. 2012. *Perspectives on Human Suffering*. Springer: Dordrecht.

Marion, J.-L. 2002. *Being Given: Toward a Phenomenology of Givenness*. Translated by J. L. Kosky. Stanford: Stanford University Press.

Sophocles. 1968. *Philoctetes*. Translated by D. Grene. In vol. 2 of *Greek Tragedies*, edited by D. Grene and R. Lattimore. Chicago: University of Chicago Press / Phoenix Books.

Palliative Care

Essential Issues

CHAPTER 8

What Is Autonomy and
What Is It Good For?

Daniel P. Sulmasy

Autonomy is widely recognized as a major (if not the primary) principle of Anglo-American bioethics. Yet one can argue that its application to clinical care, especially care at the end of life, has done more harm than good. A brief story can help to illustrate this point.

A STORY

A decade ago, while I was a Franciscan friar, I was charged with overseeing the medical care given to the friars of my province.[1] One of them, a former missionary to Bolivia whom we will call Friar Gordon, was residing in a community for retired friars in New Jersey. Outwardly gregarious but intensely private, he was a heavy smoker and hard drinker. By the time he realized he had developed lung cancer, the disease was inoperable—already metastatic to his liver and bones. He refused chemotherapy and accepted only one short course of radiation treatment before announcing that he wanted no more radiation treatment either. He had not completed a living will or health care proxy, denouncing them as worthless pieces of paper. He told his fellow friars that he did not want to be hospitalized or receive cardiopulmonary resuscitation. Fiercely independent all his life, he said he did not want hospice or even any help from the rest of the friars lest he become a burden on them. He told them what hymns he wanted at his funeral and who should preach. At first, he came regularly to community meals and evening recreation. Gradually, however, he began missing meals frequently, and they could see that he was losing weight. Next he stopped going to evening recreation and eventually stopped going to meals altogether. When the friars knocked on the door to his room to check on him, he told them, "Go away."

It was in this setting that I visited him. When I knocked on the door, I only heard a few moans in reply. I opened the door to find him lying in bed, emaciated, naked, delirious, and covered in his own feces. The room reeked. I left to fetch some clean sheets and to get the friary nurse and a couple of the friars to help me clean him up. When I asked them how they had let him get this way, and why hospice was not involved, they replied, "He said he didn't want hospice or any other form of help. We thought it was our duty to respect his autonomy."

"His autonomy!" I shouted, nearly losing it. "He's lying in his own excrement. He's your brother, not your fellow citizen. I don't care what he said. We're going to clean him up and call hospice."

AUTONOMY: THE STATUS QUO

While it is certain that this is not what the proponents of respect for patient autonomy intended, this story might illustrate a *reductio ad absurdum* refutation of the primacy given to this principle in Anglo-American bioethics. If the good of the patient is what the patient autonomously chooses even if it not what the rest would choose, this is where it leads. Something is seriously wrong with this picture. It is bioethics that has become sick. The diagnosis is *autonomia maligna*.[2]

Beauchamp and Childress, in their widely used textbook of bioethics, state simply that the principle of respect for autonomy runs as deep in the common morality as any principle of ethics.[3] In asserting this claim, these authors provide no other justification, contenting themselves to defining the term as referring to self-rule, freedom from controlling interference by others, freedom from limitations that prevent meaningful choice, and the free undertaking of acts according to a self-chosen plan.

But is it true that this concept of autonomy is, as described, a timeless and universal principle of morality? It is not historically true. The concept of autonomy does not appear in the ethical literature until Kant, and what Kant meant by autonomy was that one could not be truly free unless one's actions were in accord with the moral law.[4] That is not how most bioethicists define it today. In discussing autonomy they emphasize self-rule and freedom from external interference, not adherence to the moral law. The *Encyclopedia of Philosophy* did not even have an entry on the topic in 1969.[5] The term came to the fore in political philosophy beginning in the 1960s and was infused into bioethics some time thereafter.

It is also not transculturally true that autonomy runs deep in the common morality. Many cultures today do not regard self-rule and freedom from control by others as a fundamental principle of ethics.

Nor is it true that autonomy is an intrinsic good, so that the more autonomous one is the better a person one is. Goods like life, health, love, happiness, and peace are valuable in themselves. Autonomy is a means, not an end.

It seems reasonable, then, to ask what autonomy is good for—to ask what is good about the concept of autonomy and to demand a justification for why it should be respected if we are to get clear about its role and limits in moral thought. Failure to do any of this in bioethics has deeply afflicted our thinking about care at the end of life in perverse ways. As a consequence, Friar Gordon became a victim of *autonomia maligna*.

Despite their many protests to the contrary, autonomy dominates the bioethics of Beauchamp and Childress. They claim to have four principles: (1) autonomy, the duty to respect the preferences and self-determination of patients; (2) beneficence, the duty to advance the good of the patient; (3) nonmaleficence, the duty not to harm patients; and (4) justice, the duty to treat patients justly and to consider fairly the impact of medical decisions on others. Yet, if one peels back the onion of their system, one finds that there is really only one principle. Beneficence, for example, is defined as helping the patient; nonmaleficence as not harming the patient. Helping and not harming, however, are defined as either advancing or thwarting the interests of an individual.[6] But what makes something an interest? They define an interest as a value one autonomously chooses at a second-order level of personal reflection. That is to say, while one might prefer to undergo a fourth round of chemotherapy at a first-order level of reflection, upon deeper, second-order reflection one recognizes that one prefers chemotherapy because one has a personal interest in remaining alive, and that interest in being alive, in turn, is based on the autonomously affirmed belief that what matters most in life is being in control. Being in control is an interest. Promoting someone's interest is beneficence. Similarly, to harm someone is to thwart an interest. In the example just given, to refuse to give a fourth round of chemotherapy to the patient who prefers it would be a harm because such a refusal would wrest control away from the patient, and control is the patient's interest (i.e., her second-order autonomously chosen value). Thus, an interest is just what one really, really autonomously chooses as a value. This means, of course, that beneficence and nonmaleficence reduce to respect for autonomy. Justice similarly reduces to fairness in the distribution of opportunities to advance one's autonomously chosen preferences. In sum, the whole system thus has only one principle—autonomy—with no justification for why we ought to respect it or take it to be good.

Some have proposed a concept of relational autonomy as a correction to the perceived deficiencies of the autonomy model, but in my view the concept of relational autonomy is not a sufficient corrective. Proponents of relational autonomy still accept that "to respect autonomy is to respect each person's interests in living her life in accordance with her own conception of the good."[7] The critique they offer is that contemporary ethics does not account sufficiently for the fact that second-order preferences of certain members of society can be shaped and constrained by oppressive social relationships. While this critique is apt, the critique itself still puts autonomy at the center of ethics, arguing that we need to promote the autonomy of oppressed subjects so that they can be just as autonomous as their oppressors. The most fundamental premise remains that each is the author of his or her own conception of the good.

But can that be right? Can't one ask whether any given person's own conception of the good is correct? A theory that defines the good as a personal creation suggests that each person is a law unto herself. Yet such a theory does not seem to account sufficiently for human fallibility. We should still want to know what autonomy is and what it is good for. The failure of bioethics to even ask that question has led us into the chaotic state we find ourselves in now with respect to care at the end of life.

Beauchamp and Childress are right that autonomy has two components—liberty and agency.[8] Liberty is the external component of the concept of autonomy, concerning what one is free to do or not free to do and how one is constrained in one's choices and actions. Agency is the internal component of autonomy—the capacity for intentional action, for moral action, for choosing good or bad, and the condition for the possibility of morality itself. Agency is the supremely human but totally undifferentiated capacity for freedom of choice.

It is critical, however, to understand just how undifferentiated autonomy is. Actions are not right and good because they are freely chosen. Rather, acts are freely chosen because we think they are right and good. But we can be mistaken in our choices. Autonomy is thus not intrinsically good but the bare capacity to choose the good, the capacity for right action. It is simply a confusion and deep error in much contemporary ethical theory to regard autonomy as if it were an intrinsic good.

AUTONOMY, THE GOOD, AND THE RIGHT

The human good is not defined by autonomy but by human flourishing. The good for us is that we flourish as the kind of thing that we are—human beings. Thus, understanding the good requires us to engage in philosophical anthropology—the effort to understand what kind of thing a human being is. The word "good" is an attributive adjective, not a predicative adjective—more like the word "tall" than the word "green." To say something is tall requires that one know what kind of thing one is talking about. Similarly, to say something is good requires that one know what kind of thing one is talking about. A good human being is one that is flourishing as a human being.

What then can we say about human beings? We are complex creatures, and though it is impossible to delineate all of these complexities in a short paper, a few central features may be noted. First and foremost, we are primate mammals, but of a special sort. We are social, mutually interdependent, rational, imaginative, affective, aesthetic, spiritual beings capable of free choice, moral agency, love, humor, and grasping the finite and the infinite. Importantly, we can grasp our own finitude. We are finite physically, intellectually, and morally. These distinctive characteristics ground a moral duty to respect autonomy, as human beings are moral agents. To be a moral agent requires sufficient liberty to be able to choose the good. Human beings flourish when they freely choose the good; that is why we ought not unduly restrict human liberty.

It is instructive here to distinguish between the right and the good. The word "right" characterizes our choosing as consistent with the norms and procedures of morality, as choices conducive to human flourishing. "Good" characterizes the content of our choices when we choose states of affairs that instantiate human flourishing. Autonomy is thus not itself a good. It is the condition for the possibility of choosing the good—the condition for the possibility of moral agency. And since flourishing human beings are moral agents, it is right to promote the capacities of human beings to see themselves as moral agents capable of choosing the good. It is right to permit sufficient liberty that human beings can exercise appropriate agency. It is right to promote and encourage autonomous choices of the good. This is what respect for autonomy really means, and these are the duties that respect for autonomy ought to entail.

Yet the duty to respect autonomy, once it is understood as I have developed it, is circumscribed. One can err both in granting too much and too little liberty. To permit too little liberty restricts the flourishing of human beings by treating them paternalistically or oppressively, inhibiting the appropriate exercise of their agency. To permit too much liberty, however, can also be wrong, restricting human flourishing by failing to help shape the agency of human beings toward the good. Societies that err in this way can be characterized as licentious. Individuals that err in this way can be characterized as indifferent. To say, "Do whatever you want. It's none of my business" is not respectful. If we truly respect the autonomy of human beings for the right reasons, we do so because we want them to flourish by using their agency to choose the good. We can, therefore, err morally by either granting too much or too little liberty. Friar Gordon had not chosen the good. He was not flourishing. Respecting his liberty was not respectful of him as a moral agent, not respectful of his dignity.

Human beings ought to be accorded wide, but not absolute, liberty. The primary reason that we need to grant wide berth to human choice is that the good for human beings is pluralistic, not monistic. This is true for several reasons that are especially salient in health care. First, human beings are constitutively diverse. Humans are genetically, epigenetically, physically diverse. Diseases differ. Pain thresholds differ. Responses to drugs differ. Individuals are typically better judges of their physical status than others.

Second, human beings are subject to both natural and social lotteries. Where one was born, into what culture, what economy, what legal system, what family all contribute to plurality in the human good.

Third, human beings have narrative histories. While it is not true that we make ourselves, we are shaped by our choices and the choices of others. Human lives traverse unique historical arcs.

Fourth, the states that constitute human good are plural. There is not one human good, such as pleasure. Moreover, somewhat paradoxically, the free exercise of agency always restricts liberty. To choose one thing is not to choose something else. Agency is exercised in finitude. There are many potential human goods, and no one can choose them all. For example, to pursue musical excellence may mean forgoing athletic endeavors. Or, as a patient of mine just recently related to me, a choice to move from the West Coast to the East Coast for the good of an ailing wife meant forgoing major career goals. The exercise of agency delimits liberty and constrains other choices.

Finally, freedom is future-oriented. Human agency renders us open to possibility, open to growth and change. All of this means that the human good is incredibly diverse. What is good for one human being is not good for another. Our duty is to permit sufficient agency for human beings to flourish pluralistically. The ethical naturalism for which I am arguing must be liberal in this sense.

This pluralism with respect to the good is not, however, a form of moral subjectivism. There will be a set of choices that are clearly inconsistent with human flourishing and wrong for all human beings. There will be choices that are objectively good for particular individuals even if they are not good for others, given that each human being is a unique event in history. To understand the good as particular does not imply moral subjectivism.

Yet, as I have argued, unbridled liberty is also an ethical mistake. That the good is plural does not entail that each individual is a law unto herself. Good societies have an obligation to restrict liberty that goes beyond Mill's harm principle. The nineteenth-century philosopher John Stuart Mill holds the view that liberty must be respected because self-determination is an intrinsic good, and liberty can only be restricted when one's choice harms others.[9] That is to say, for Mill, being free from the controlling influences of others and being the self-determining agent of one's life is intrinsically good, and neither the state nor the medical profession ought to limit one's liberty unless what one proposes to do harms others or limits the liberty of others. The Millian view, however, is unduly broad, suffering from confusion about the nature of human liberty, agency, and the human good. As I have explained, the goal of respecting autonomy is not to allow each to define the good for himself but to allow sufficient liberty to permit the individual and his society to flourish through the free choice of the good. Freedom is not intrinsically good but the opportunity to do good, the opportunity to act rightly or wrongly. The good is not simply what we choose to call good or what we assert is good for us. The good depends upon an objective understanding of the kinds of things that human beings are. Thus, choices that undermine or contradict human dignity, or acts that could not be under any circumstances construed as consistent with human flourishing, can, and should, be restricted.

Likewise, choices that undermine or contradict the flourishing of others with whom one is in constitutive relationship as a social being can, and should, be prohibited. Some rules of thumb can be offered to help clarify these restrictions further. First, greater deference should be given to what are typically called negative rights than to positive rights. An individual's claim to the autonomy to refuse having something done to her is greater than her claim to have something done for her. Second, flourishing for human beings is both individual and social. Human beings are inherently social. Attempts to promote the flourishing of individuals by restricting their liberty ought not do net harm to the common good. This is a principle that dates to Thomas of Aquinas.[10] Third, attempts to enhance the flourishing of human beings by promoting choices for the good ought not to do so at the expense of their agency. The "nudges" of so-called libertarian paternalism tend dangerously in this direction. Human beings are not really flourishing if their choices of the good are not truly free.

These are rules of thumb not for determining what is right or wrong but for determining what restrictions a society can place on the liberty of human beings to make morally right or wrong decisions. Not all morally wrong actions can, or should, be prohibited by law.

IMPLICATIONS FOR CARE AT THE END OF LIFE

So, what does all this mean for autonomy and care at the end of life?

1. Forgoing Burdensome and/or Nonbeneficial Treatments

We need to recognize the physical finitude of human beings if we are to make choices that help patients to flourish as the kind of things that they are—finite human beings. Choices to forgo life-sustaining treatments are consistent with human flourishing. To continue treatment past the point of reasonability can be a denial of the reality of human physical finitude and inconsistent with human flourishing. Attempts at cardiopulmonary resuscitation in patients with untreatable metastatic cancer typically fall in this category.

Nonetheless, we will need to recognize a plurality of choices regarding when to stop treatment and when to continue treatment, consistent with the plurality of the human good. The choice to take another round of chemotherapy to extend life a few weeks in order to see a child get married will be right for some and wrong for others. But the standard for judging the validity of a request would shift from the bare fact that it was autonomously made to how that choice would contribute to individual and communal human flourishing. That shift seems subtle, but it would be monumental.

2. Palliating Symptoms and Addressing Suffering

The palliation of symptoms can be seen as a way of restoring agency to dying persons as well as a direct bestowing of the intrinsic good of symptom control. Palliation ought thus to be seen as a moral duty. It eases the suffering of the dying, instantiates the virtue of compassion in caregivers, and contributes to our flourishing as finite creatures. Additionally, we will need to recognize opportunities for growth at the end of life—psychological, spiritual, and even intellectual growth. Human freedom is oriented to the future, to possibility, to hope. Dying persons are still human beings who can flourish as they are dying, growing as persons and teaching the rest of us who survive them lessons about life and its meaning.

3. The Limits of Liberty at the End of Life

Importantly, some choices can and should be prohibited as inconsistent with human flourishing, individual or collective. This would include choices that undermine the intrinsic human dignity that is the basis of morality itself or undermine our individual and collective flourishing as the kinds of things that we are. The point of liberty, after all, is to enhance human agency, and the elimination of agency in the name of liberty is not genuine autonomy. Assisted suicide and euthanasia would thus be among the prohibited choices.

Human autonomy is not atomistic and individualistic but interrelational and communal. The liberty that promotes the human agent's capacity to choose the good promotes choices that are for others.

CONCLUSION

So, what is autonomy for? It is for others.

Friar Gordon had lived most of his life, admirably, as a missionary serving others freely. When he was dying, however, and could no longer freely choose to serve others and could no longer live independently, he did not thereby cease to be fully human or lose his intrinsic human dignity. What he needed to learn at that moment of his life was how to receive freely from others. In failing to do so, he prevented himself from flourishing, even as a dying person, to the fullest extent possible, even in the face of the limitation and suffering illness will inevitably impose on each of us. Compounding matters, those caring for him mistakenly believed that his previously expressed autonomous preferences not to receive the help of others should, as a matter of ethics, guide his care. This mistaken version of ethics (so popular in today's bioethics) resulted in treatment that was actually inhumane, caused Friar Gordon even greater suffering, and frustrated the possibilities for his flourishing in the face of death.

Friar Gordon's autonomous preferences were clearly and objectively at odds with his flourishing. When one understands respect for autonomy as the need to give others the liberty they need to be able to choose the good and to flourish as the kinds of things that they are, one is liberated, as a caregiver, from slavish obedience to the constraints imposed by the autonomous choices of others that frustrate their own ability to flourish. His caregivers could have been liberated to care genuinely for Friar Gordon, bathing him, feeding him, treating his symptoms, praying with him (and for him) as a fellow human being whose value rests in his humanity and not in his mistaken choices.

We flourish most when we choose to love and can flourish in and through the process of dying by choosing to die virtuously. For Christians, this involves the supernatural virtues of faith, hope, and love. Christians hold these virtues to be God-given gifts that allow persons to move beyond themselves into the communion of saints. To die in faith, hope, and love is to know the freedom of the children of God. That's the point of autonomy. Love is not love unless it's free. And the disposition of our liberty that is required by the exercise of agency for the sake of love is the only road to true freedom. The human being fully alive and integrally flourishing as a full-standing member of the human community faces death with the freedom that love alone makes possible. Palliative care has the opportunity to remind the rest of contemporary Western medicine of this important truth.

NOTES

1. I was formally released from vows in 2011 and have been happily married for nearly a decade.

2. I first heard this phrase in a private conversation with Professor Patricia Marshall.

3. Beauchamp and Childress 2012, 101.

4. Kant 2002.

5. Edwards 1967.

6. Beauchamp and Childress 2012, 153–54, 182.

7. Mackenzie 2008, 512.

8. Beauchamp and Childress 2012, 102.

9. Mill 2003.

10. Thomas of Aquinas 1964, II-I; II-II.

WORKS CITED

Beauchamp, T., and J. Childress. 2012. *Principles of Biomedical Ethics.* New York: Oxford University Press.

Edwards, P., ed. 1967. *The Encyclopedia of Philosophy.* New York: Macmillan.

Kant, I. 2002. *Groundwork on the Metaphysics of Morals.* Edited by A. Wood and J. Schneewind. New Haven: Yale University Press.

Mackenzie, C. 2008. "Relational Autonomy, Normative Authority and Perfectionism." *Journal of Social Philosophy* 39 (4): 512–33.

Mill, J. S. 2003. *On Liberty.* Edited by D. Bromwich, J. B. Elshtain, and G. Kateb. New Haven: Yale University Press.

Thomas of Aquinas. 1964. *Summa Theologiae.* Blackfriars edition. Edited by T. Gilby and T. C. O'Brien. New York: McGraw-Hill.

CHAPTER 9

Human Flourishing and Palliative Care

Autonomy, Mortality, and Rationality

Robin W. Lovin

The cases are familiar. Mrs. Smith, a woman in her early eighties, has suffered a stroke that left her partly paralyzed and often somewhat confused. She has not made progress with physical therapy, and it is becoming clear that her care will now involve managing several permanently debilitating conditions. Mr. Kim, a man in his sixties, has cancer. Further treatment is unlikely to limit its spread and will only aggravate the painful complications of his earlier surgery and chemotherapy. He is about to return home, where friends and family seem determined to give him the sense of a return to normal life, even though none of them knows quite what to expect next. Mrs. Rodriguez has survived an acute respiratory infection and is ready to return to the nursing home, where she will receive help with the advanced Parkinson's disease that leaves her unable to care for herself. She seems depressed.

Each of these patients is at the point of transition from an effort at cure to a plan designed to manage serious, ongoing limitations, control pain, and sustain quality of life. Each case deserves the best medical knowledge, clinical skills, and sympathetic attention from physicians and other caregivers. But the cases may not seem to raise any of the familiar problems of medical ethics. There are no scarce resources to be allocated here, no experimental treatments for which risks must be weighed against possible benefits, and no immediate questions about terminating treatment to allow an imminent, natural death. These cases are hard work, but it seems they largely avoid the hard questions.

Nevertheless, the transition to palliative care engages questions of ethics at the most basic level. To make decisions about a course of treatment when disease is chronic, impairments are irreversible, and death may be expected in months requires patients, families, and medical professionals to ask what makes for a good human life, what is the best combination of human goods that can be achieved under present circumstances, how to respect the needs, desires, and competences of everyone involved, and how to relate a good life now to a good life as a whole.

What makes these questions basic to ethics is that in one way or another, all of us are confronted with them all the time, whatever our situation may be. More difficult questions raise interesting problems about when and whether it is permissible to do some particular harm to achieve some good or about how to allocate burdens fairly in a bad situation. Special cases like the classic "trolley problem"[1] occupy ethics classes for hours because they seem unresolvable. But the questions that arise in palliative care are engaging because they are so *familiar*. To make the best use of our circumstances, to recognize the limits of our possibilities, and to focus attention on our most important goals are challenges we all face. The problems of palliative care illuminate the moral life for everyone because palliative care is continuous with the wider moral life. It involves making choices about conditions that are basic to human nature and integral to human flourishing. In this discussion, we will focus on two of these in particular: mortality and autonomy. These are, of course, basic concerns in all decisions about patient care, but considering them as human goods will help us to see how the problems of palliative care can lead us to think more broadly about medicine and the moral life.

QUESTIONS OF ETHICS

People have many different ways of talking about ethics. They speak in terms of commandments and prohibitions. They elaborate systems of rules, identify virtues, and balance rights and duties. Many different sources—theology, tradition, law, wisdom, expertise, or power—may be identified as the origin of these ideas, but all of them provide understandings of the human person against which judgments and actions can be measured. Right actions and good judgments align with this idea of human nature and lead to the flourishing of the persons with whom we are concerned. Wrong choices contradict human nature and lead to various problems that result from expecting something more, or less, or at least different from what the human person is constituted to do and to be.

The Real Goods with Which Ethics Begins

The idea that moral systems are grounded in a normative human nature is variously called "moral realism" or "ethical naturalism" or even "natural law" ethics. There are alternatives to this way of thinking about ethics, of course, but human nature is a kind of intuitive starting point around which we can organize a discussion of the aims of the moral life. In the Western tradition, the idea goes back at least to Aristotle, who suggested that life lived in accordance with human nature leads to *eudaimonia*.[2] The word may be translated as "happiness," but it also implies deeper notions of fulfillment or satisfaction suggested by the phrase "human flourishing." Recent philosophers following in this broadly Aristotelian way of thinking have also spoken of a "human capabilities" approach, arguing that a good life involves realizing, for oneself and others, the possibilities inherent in human nature.[3]

The study of ethics thus involves identifying goods that human beings need to live well, separating these real goods from contingent and passing desires, and ordering the real goods in sustainable constellations that make it possible to attain other goods in the future. Human nature requires food and shelter, freedom from fear and pain, and the support of a community that provides order, security, and subsistence. The goods of friendship also flourish in this environment, particularly if a person has enough leisure to appreciate them, and Aristotle supposes that under these conditions the pleasures of knowledge, understanding, and contemplation will also follow in due course. This is a high standard for "happiness," and Aristotle's writings on ethics seem to assume that only a small minority will have the resources to achieve it. Others—women, slaves, and foreigners, for example—are not active participants in the *politea*, the moral community that centers on the political life of the city. Aristotle's politics may strike us as antiquated or even offensive, but his basic way of thinking that identifies and orders goods is common to human experience, and we all use it when we choose more difficult and more durable goals over immediate satisfactions. Aristotle is surely right that understanding the highest good is what enables us to order the lower ones, and an important part of human flourishing is knowing what is still worth choosing when the best is not available. If Aristotle focused rather narrowly on achieving the best possible life, we can also turn his way of identifying and ordering human goods toward achieving the best life possible. *To be concerned with achieving the good under less than ideal conditions describes the moral life for most of us. It is, especially, what palliative care specialists do.*

Seeking Real Goods Is the Center of the Moral Life

The persistence of Aristotelian moral realism through the history of Western ethics suggests the flexibility and adaptiveness of this way of thinking. Similar lines of thought appear in other literatures and cultures, including Confucian and Taoist accounts of virtue and a variety of creation narratives that link moral expectations to the conditions under which human nature was formed.[4] These traditions do not agree on their accounts of human flourishing, even within themselves. But they point to a nearly universal way of thinking about the realization of human purposes by individuals and societies. *Our life is oriented to achieve its needs within a framework provided by the order of nature and the legacies of previous human efforts, and it draws meaning from contemplation of ourselves in relation to reality as whole.* These achievements are difficult and fragile, and they depend more on circumstances and luck than Aristotle thought they did.[5] Our ideas about human good must be reconsidered in response to successes and failures, our own and others', but they are not simply products of our desires or flights of imagination. Human goods are realities to be known, and knowing them bends the will toward their realization. When the effort succeeds, we flourish.

FROM REAL GOODS TO MORAL RULES

If this reflection on goods and virtues seems unlike the codes of ethics, case studies, and decision-making procedures that accompany most discussions of medical ethics, that is because ethics in an institutional setting usually operates at some distance from the questions about human nature and human flourishing that might occupy a moral theorist who is thinking in the terms we have just reviewed. Organizations usually codify their thinking about ethics in general rules, which can be impartially applied and determine choices apart from individual judgments about the good. Especially in institutional settings, where the people involved probably hold a variety of incompatible ideas about the good, a very "thin" theory about the most basic human goods may provide a starting point, but contested choices have to be made according to agreed rules.[6] Where goods do figure in decision-making, they must be of the most general sort, avoiding precisely the sort of choices between different goods that figure so prominently in individual lives. Maximizing wealth or lifting broad indices of "general welfare" provides the criteria for public choices, with the assumption that individuals will be free to make use of the resources thus provided to put together their own good lives according to their own ideas.

Why Medicine Needs Rules

Medicine typically encounters ethics in these discussions that take place at some distance from the basic questions of human flourishing. Protocols for decision-making, rules about consultation and disclosure, considerations of public health, and prohibitions against certain actions are the daily substance of medical ethics. Their purpose often seems to be setting a limit on reflection about particular human goods, lest someone be tempted to achieve their own preferred good at an unacceptable cost. The ancient injunction "First, do no harm" still provides the most general rule in a system that relies more on rules than on goods and virtues.

This in itself reflects the realities of human life and the institutional constraints of medical practice. Life and health are among the most basic human goods, and while they are uncertain by nature, people at least want clear expectations about what those who take these goods into their hands are going to do. Medical professionals must react quickly, and patients are often drawn unexpectedly into the system, without opportunity to reflect on what they might want as the outcome. A system of rules, formulated and applied by impartial reason, serves the practice of medicine well. A reflection on the more basic questions of ethics might well conclude that, given the biological constraints of human life and the complexity of the institutional structures needed for the practice of modern medicine, such rules are among the goods that human flourishing requires. But even when we are confident that we have followed the rules and that the rules we have followed are good ones, we might well ask whether we have done enough for Mrs. Smith, Mr. Kim, and Mrs. Rodriguez.

Why Rules Are Not Enough

This is because, in medicine as in life, our moral concerns cannot be reduced to a system of rules. At the most basic level, ethics remains a question of specific human goods, how these goods are related to one another in a good life, and what personal characteristics or virtues will sustain that life. General goods like health must be analyzed into particular human goods, such as relief from pain, freedom of movement, the enjoyment of personal relationships, or making one's own choices. Each of these goods must be understood in its particularity, with the understanding that human goods are largely incommensurable. That is, we cannot simply equate this much personal relationship with that much freedom from pain, so much enjoyment of daily activities with so much meaningful work, this much quality of life with that much length of it. Each of these goods must be understood in its specific forms and then balanced against other goods in an assessment of what human flourishing means under present and possible future conditions. There is no algorithm for this and no common scale against which all these goods can be measured. It is a decision that human beings must make about human goods. That is, it is a moral judgment.[7]

In palliative care, medicine returns to ethics at this most basic level. Rules and protocols are important because medicine is a risky business that requires the coordination of actions and expectations between many people in a short time frame. But deciding on a course of care when both medicine and life are at their limits involves detailed judgments about human goods and balancing them in a whole human life. When some generalized ideal of physical and mental health is no longer possible, it becomes important to identify the individual elements of human flourishing, determine the ways in which they are each still available, and consider how they may be related in what is still recognizably a good life, especially for the patient but also for others who are closely connected with this life.

Of course, not all human goods are equally relevant to palliative care. Full exercise of one's highest abilities was part of Aristotle's definition of *eudaimonia*, and the realization of lifelong ambitions remains important even at the end of life. But there are things that can no longer be done. Even when creative and analytical abilities remain strong, strength and concentration required to complete a sustained work may be lacking. Mrs. Rodriguez may have devoted her retirement years to a community garden project or especially enjoyed sharing dinners with her extended family and afternoon card games with her friends. The projects and relationships constructed over decades remain valuable, even if they cannot be continued in the same way. To speak of a good life at the end of life is not about humoring the patient or raising expectations that cannot be met. But neither is it simply a matter of minimizing discomfort and accepting limitations. Palliative care recognizes specific goods that human nature will still support and recasts durable goals to fit existing conditions. Mrs. Rodriguez may never turn her spade in the community garden again, but she might, even with some discomfort—and some inconvenience to her caregivers—be able to visit the garden and talk with the people with whom she shared it. Nor should these occasions be devoted solely to remembrance of times past. There is value in seeing that the work goes on, meeting new people who are involved with it, and envisioning what the garden will be like when she is no longer around to see it. A good life for Mrs. Rodriguez involves sharing these experiences with others and incorporating them into her new situation.

MORTALITY AND AUTONOMY AS HUMAN GOODS

Palliative care moves first to relieve physical and mental suffering, but as we gain control of those problems, we can begin to consider the specific human goods that remain relevant to each individual patient. In this brief essay, we can only illustrate the possibilities with an overview of the goods related to two important aspects of human nature: mortality and autonomy. These are durable features of individual and social life, and they are particularly relevant to the ways that medical professionals become involved in decisions about palliative care.

Mortality: The Human Good at the End of Life

It may seem strange to include mortality in a discussion of human goods, but that is a reminder that behind the rules and principles, ethics is about a good life within the limits of human nature. The modern preference to ignore death and postpone recognition of aging is a denial of the human good rather than a way of achieving it. It is a dualistic view, in which the search for a good life ends when the process of dying begins. Sometimes, too, resistance to recognizing mortality takes the form of skepticism about palliative care itself. Those who focus on medicine at the end of life are considered perhaps too quick to give up on the possibilities for cure, or even suspected of aiming to bring difficult lives to a premature end. Moral realism, by contrast, seeks to include a good death in its account of human flourishing.

Death, of course, is inevitable. But the end of life is, as some theologians have said, a *finis*, not a *telos*.[8] It is an end in the sense of a stop but not an end in the sense of a goal. So the question human nature poses is how to manage these inevitabilities. Often this leads to a foreshortening of perspective, so that we focus on whether a person has a good life under present conditions or whether a person has a good "quality of life" in relation to his or her present capabilities. The question about human flourishing and human mortality should be put in another way. *We seek to care for a person at the end of life in such a way that when the* finis *is reached, we will say that the ending was consistent with the good life in accord with human nature that was the* telos *through the whole of life.*

Mr. Kim, the cancer patient whose disease with its complications must now be seen as terminal, will return home on a palliative plan of care. It may be some time before he and his caregivers have to consider withdrawing treatment altogether and allowing a natural death to occur. Care for Mr. Kim involves more than keeping him comfortable and waiting for the inevitable end. It may involve resuming his normal activities at a level appropriate to his strength and interest. But it also involves a clear-sighted recognition that he is entering the last phase of his life, however long that may be. He needs opportunities for relationships and reconciliations that may be at odds with simply avoiding discomfort. He needs to dispose of his assets and possessions in ways that bring a life's work to a conclusion. This may be done in symbolic ways with important objects and small gifts, of course, or it may involve the implementation of estate plans made long in advance. But it requires a level of attentiveness on the part of the patient that may require medical support, and those who have been part of his life and can be gathered must be more than recipients of bequests. We bring a life to a *telos* by hearing stories or by retelling them, if the dying person cannot do it themself. All this requires a recognition of mortality that perhaps comes earlier than a treatment program that simply anticipates the final stages of Mr. Kim's illness might suggest, and it may require a level of consciousness that cannot be achieved if the only goals are to control pain and maintain the semblance of a normal life. The range of human goods available to Mr. Kim in his final illness may seem narrow compared to those achievable in its prime, but bringing life to a *telos*, rather than merely waiting for the end, requires understanding those goods in their specificity and balancing them in an act of moral judgment.

Autonomy: Enabling Choices as Well as Respecting Them

A critic might observe that "bringing life to a *telos*" suggests the perspective of an external observer who is evaluating the end of a life rather than the experience of the person living it. Even the idea that we are in a position to judge what is a "good death" raises questions about how understanding mortality relates to autonomy, the second aspect of human nature that we are considering as part of our understanding of palliative care.

Mrs. Rodriguez has survived an acute respiratory infection, but her Parkinson's disease is chronic and requires her return to a nursing home, where her opportunities to make decisions about the course of her life, her daily activities, and even her immediate bodily needs may be severely limited. The human goods she lacks are not just the things she might seek if she were able but the more basic capacity to make decisions about her own life. That capacity is itself a human good, which cannot be replaced simply by being handed good things that others have chosen for us.

Autonomy is the possibility of choosing a course of action, instead of being coerced by others or driven by one's own fears and desires. As the Greek roots of autonomy imply, we are *auto-nomos* when we give ourselves a *nomos*, a law or a rule, rather than following somebody else's rule or being ruled by our passions. While the origins of the term are ancient, it has a key role in modern thought beginning with the work of Immanuel Kant (1724–1804).[9] For Kant, autonomy was central to moral decisions. To do the right thing simply at the direction of another, without the application of one's own reason, is not a moral act at all. Nor is a goal that is simply the object of desire a real human good. In the two centuries since Kant wrote, autonomy has become central to our understanding of political rights, personal freedom, and medical ethics.[10]

The problem is that, while a capacity for autonomy is part of human nature, autonomy itself is an achievement. We tend to see it as a personal achievement, especially at the beginning of life, as a child becomes a distinct, unique person, capable of taking responsibility for his or her actions.[11] But in dealing with medical cases, we realize that autonomy is also a social achievement, especially at the end of life and in extreme conditions. A person like Mrs. Rodriguez, depressed by the limitations imposed by chronic illness, is not autonomous, even if her physician has fully informed her about her condition and the choices it requires. Indeed, being fully informed may leave her feeling less able to make a choice.

The medical professions make autonomy possible by alleviating pain, fear, and other forms of distress. But they also promote autonomy by helping patients understand their condition and possible responses to the condition. If the goal is autonomy, the decisions that we would want to help a patient consider extend beyond treatment options and may involve a wide range of caregiver interactions. For Mrs. Rodriguez, autonomy may depend on making sure that she has opportunities to interact with people from outside the nursing home environment. It may also involve a critical look at procedures and staffing in that environment, as well as reconsidering options at other care facilities or for home care. Each of those steps can be regarded as a part of respect for patient autonomy, even if they go well beyond the usual planning for a course of treatment and involve family members, religious communities, social workers, and financial planners in the process along with the medical team. The patient's autonomy is expanded, not diminished, as more people become involved in the choices.

One way to define the scope of palliative care, then, is to calibrate it, not against the symptoms of distress, but against the requirements of human flourishing. Palliative care recognizes autonomy, but it is also concerned to enable it, sustain it, and even, if possible, to restore it when pain and diminished capacities have taken it away.

REAL GOODS AND REAL CHOICES

Our consideration of mortality and autonomy thus leads away from guidance that can easily be formulated in rules and protocols and back toward ideas about human nature and human good that have been central to moral thinking throughout history. *Palliative care engages these basic questions of ethics precisely because it is concerned with how a person flourishes within the given conditions of life.* Goods one might consider in health are genuinely different from those considered in the most serious illness when palliative care is sought. These different goods must be understood in their specificity and balanced in such a way that the result is recognizably a good life for the person concerned.

Human Goods Are Social Achievements

Engaging these basic questions of ethics as they arise in the lives of patients like Mrs. Smith, Mr. Kim, and Mrs. Rodriguez leads us to rethink the dimensions of palliative care, expanding it to include all aspects of a patient's life, rather than limiting it to questions of how to control pain, live with disabilities, or manage treatment at the end of life. But if the questions of ethics change the way we think about palliative care, the problems of palliative care also change the way we think about ethics. It is an important theoretical exercise to envision a good life, as Aristotle did, in terms of the highest goods achievable by persons gifted with ample resources, good education, and a bit of luck. But the real questions of ethics are usually about the best combination of real goods that can be achieved by people working together under real limitations. Decisions about palliative care thus remind us of something that modern individualism often forgets: human goods are in important ways *social* achievements. Even personal virtues require a social infrastructure that makes individual discernment and discipline possible. That is why the most important classical virtues of prudence, courage, temperance, and justice are oriented toward fitting a good person for life in a good society. *Especially when we seek the good of persons whose lives are limited, fragile, and perhaps short, flourishing depends on the collaboration of many people and on effective coordination of their efforts.* This poses a risk of paternalism, especially for the professionals who are in charge of the coordination, but it is a risk that must be run.

Palliative Care, Medical Science, and Human Goods

We find ourselves at a point in modern medicine and in modern life where we must begin to question the goals of medicine taught in scientific terms alone.

From the beginning of the modern era, growing scientific knowledge of the causes and courses of disease has led to ever more complex, aggressive, and effective ways of treating them. The benefits of this scientific rationality are obvious. It expands autonomy and can hold mortality at bay. Diseases that once killed thousands now are virtually unknown. Surgical procedures that once were risky are now routine and often are on their way to being replaced in turn by nanotechnologies that are less invasive and promise even less risk. We are not only less susceptible to the sudden experience of a bad death than our ancestors were. We are significantly more autonomous than those who lived their lives in anticipation of a yearly outbreak of yellow fever or the prospect that this winter's cold might develop into fatal pneumonia. But medicine has often been discussed and taught as if cure were the only purpose of our interventions, as if that goal were worth any cost, and as if any other outcome were a failure.

Perhaps, then, as we consider such ordinary cases as the stroke patient whose life is suddenly limited, the cancer patient whose condition no longer holds a realistic hope for cure, and the nursing home patient who can no longer make simple decisions for herself, we get a different perspective on what it means to promote the good of the patient. With a return to the most basic questions of ethics, we can see the emergence of palliative care not as a new subspecialty for cases that do not, for the moment, respond to our efforts at cure, but as a new paradigm for medicine, and perhaps for science more generally. That paradigm would see progress taking place within limits set by personal mortality and planetary fragility, and it focuses on human goods to enable us to choose the things we value within those limits. By reconnecting medical ethics with this broader framework of moral reasoning, palliative care provides a paradigm that is less about means and ends and more about locating those ends within a range of human possibilities. Precisely because this new paradigm recognizes that human beings cannot have all they want of everything they want, it judges that a rational outcome depends in large part on a hard look at the balance between competing goods that results from the choices made within limits.

Thinking about the interaction of mortality, autonomy, and medical science in pursuit of a good human life (and death as part of life) helps us see an important transformation in thinking that takes place as palliative care becomes central to medicine. It began, perhaps, with the greater emphasis on autonomy that gave the patient a greater role in choosing outcomes, even when that outcome was not identical with the technical goal of medical practice. But we have learned rather quickly that, although autonomy is always to be respected, it is not easily achieved. Health, autonomy, and even mortality are social conditions that are brought about and sustained in our dealings with one another. We are still far from a complete understanding of how these multiple possibilities and ultimate limits interact in the future of humanity and the future of the planet. But we work together daily on the task of connecting mortality, autonomy, and our common humanity for ourselves and for those within our care.

NOTES

1. Thomson 1985. The dilemma is whether we should save the lives of five people who will be killed by a runaway trolley by diverting it so that as a result of our intervention one person will be killed. The variations on the problem are numerous.
2. Aristotle 2000, 10.
3. Nussbaum 2011.
4. Lovin and Reynolds 1985.
5. Nussbaum 2001.
6. Rawls 1971, 395–99.
7. Cf. Aristotle 2000, 4–5.
8. Moltmann 2002.
9. Kant 1997.
10. Beauchamp and Childress 2001, 57–112.
11. Erikson 1964, 118–20.

WORKS CITED

Aristotle. 2000. *Nicomachean Ethics.* Edited by R. Crisp. Cambridge: Cambridge University Press.

Beauchamp, T., and J. Childress. 2001. *Principles of Biomedical Ethics.* 5th ed. New York: Oxford University Press.

Erikson, E. 1964. *Insight and Responsibility.* New York: W. W. Norton.

Kant, I. 1997 [1785]. *Groundwork of the Metaphysics of Morals.* Edited by M. Gregor. Cambridge: Cambridge University Press.

Lovin, R. W., and F. E. Reynolds, eds. 1985. *Cosmogony and Ethical Order.* Chicago: University of Chicago Press.

Moltmann, J. 2002. "The End as Beginning." *Word and World* 22 (3): 221–27.

Nussbaum, M. 2001. *The Fragility of Goodness: Luck and Ethics in Greek Tragedy and Philosophy.* Rev. ed. Cambridge: Cambridge University Press.

———. 2011. *Creating Capabilities: The Human Development Approach.* Cambridge, MA: Belknap Press.

Rawls, J. 1971. *A Theory of Justice.* Cambridge, MA: Harvard University Press.

Thomson, J. J. 1985. "The Trolley Problem." *Yale Law Journal* 94 (6): 1395–415.

CHAPTER 10

The Robin Hood of Opioids

Palliative Care in the Underdeveloped World

James Cleary

I first met Artur in Ukraine, during one of the coldest winters I have ever experienced. I had practiced palliative medicine in Wisconsin for years, and I thought I knew winter cold. However, Wisconsin winters had not prepared me for Ukrainian winter, any more than my practice of palliative medicine at the University of Wisconsin had prepared me for palliative medicine in Ukraine. I quickly realized it was not only the winter that was brutal in Ukraine.

Artur, a former KGB colonel, was living with prostate cancer, metastatic to bone. His pain was often so intense he could not move. He had self-isolated from his family in Kiev to a small dacha a few hours away because he "did not want them to see me cry." On his small snow-covered farm, Artur did as well as he could, keeping the wood fire burning, preparing small meals, and caring for his livestock when able. His ability to move was dictated by uneven access to pain relief. No strong oral pain medicine was available. If lucky, a nurse would come four times a day to give him a morphine injection. If unlucky, then more pain. But even on his lucky days there was not enough pain relief, and so Artur shared with me his other solutions.

The first was drinking a bottle of brandy daily. After downing one of his many brandies and while holding an honorary citation from President Gorbachev acknowledging his wartime service in Afghanistan, he shared his other solution. He reached across the bed on which he was sitting and produced from under the pillows the service revolver that he kept loaded "for when the pain gets too bad!" There was no warning for this action, and I was taken aback, no, shocked, to see him waving the gun through the air, even though he was not holding it as if to shoot. But still, it was a gun!

What was I, a native of balmy Australia, a palliative care physician and professor of medicine at the University of Wisconsin and director of the Pain and Policy Studies Group (PPSG), a WHO-collaborating center for pain policy and palliative care, doing in this situation in the middle of winter in rural Ukraine? I had been invited to participate in a film documentary project with three master's-level journalism students from the University of British Columbia, together with a faculty producer/videographer, a driver, and a Ukrainian interpreter. The students' class had chosen the international lack of access to pain relief outside of the most-developed countries as the topic of their master's project and had sent film crews to India, Uganda, and Ukraine. With the help of palliative care advocates in each country, they had identified people willing to share their stories about living with pain in the absence of adequate access to morphine and other opioids, something most citizens in the developed world do not experience.

Morphine is the foundational opioid and an essential medicine for both acute and chronic cancer pain relief as well as many other conditions causing serious pain. Amazingly, 80 percent of the world's population lacks access to morphine—a frightening inequity.[1] Ukraine is but one of many countries without adequate access,[2] as I witnessed firsthand with Artur. In his case, there was some access to morphine. But unlike in North America and most other European countries, where morphine can be prescribed, dispensed, and taken by patients as a tablet (both short and long acting), morphine in Ukraine was only available as an injection administered by a nurse visiting his home four times daily, if the nurse's schedule and the weather allowed. Yet even on a good day, injectable morphine typically relieved pain for three to four hours, leaving a patient like Artur with unrelieved pain for a third to a half of every day.

Artur's situation was not unique. We visited a local hospital where cancer patients were receiving regular injections of morphine, providing at least temporarily adequate pain relief. But there, a treating physician shared her moral distress in knowing the great suffering her cancer patients would experience after discharge through the lack of home access to pain medicines. We also spoke to the mother of a brain tumor patient, Vlad, whose pain was so severe, even in the hospital, that he had attempted to end his life by throwing himself out of a hospital window rather than live with the severe and constant pain of his incurable brain cancer. Vlad's mother shared photos and stories of Vlad, and we accompanied her to the church where she prayed for the soul of her now-deceased son. "Why couldn't he have had pain relief?" she continued to ask. "Why did he have to suffer?"

Indeed, why couldn't Vlad or Artur or innumerable patients like them across the planet count on adequate pain relief, especially in the setting of serious or terminal illness? While suicide may not be on the minds of all those facing the undertreatment of cancer pain, the unbearable suffering of many around the world is a shocking reality. With the increasing control of most infectious diseases, cancer and other noncommunicable diseases such as heart and lung disease have become the leading causes of death, not just in high-income countries but also in low- and middle-income countries.[3] And the health care systems, or lack thereof, result in the majority of cancer patients presenting with advanced disease, particularly of the liver, the lung, and, in women, the cervix. Palliative care and pain relief is absolutely critical for these patients and should include access to morphine and other opioids (narcotics) to ensure some degree of comfort. But the benefits of these medicines are not available to most of the world's population.

A HISTORY OF MEDICAL OPIOID USE AND REGULATION

Historically, the products of the poppy have been used for centuries to bring about pain relief. The Greco-Roman physician Dioscorides wrote of this property in his work *De materia medica* in the first century. Morphine, chemically identified in the early nineteenth century, became widely used for acute pain during the US Civil War, following the advent of the hypodermic needle. Heroin was synthesized in the late nineteenth century and marketed as a cough suppressant with reportedly less addiction than morphine.

The expansion of morphine's use for cancer pain grew through hospices, primarily hospices associated with religious organizations. When Dr. Cicely Saunders reported the regular use of morphine for improved pain control in London hospice patients, she was documenting the work of nuns at St. Joseph's Hospice. While the traditional orders in the early 1920s were for half to one grain (30 to 60 mg) of morphine to be administered orally every four hours "as needed," these nuns decided "as needed" should be interpreted as strictly every four hours to ensure patient comfort. This practice, published early in Dr. Saunders's medical career, showed that the regular administration of morphine resulted in improved pain control.[4]

With the start of St. Christopher's Hospice in England in the early 1960s, considerable focus was given to improving pain relief, with research being done on the use of morphine and heroin for pain control. Concurrently, access to opioids was being considered by the United Nations. The 1961 Single Convention on Narcotic Drugs established that opioids (narcotics) should be available for medical and scientific purposes while reducing the risk of misuse and diversion took place.[5] However, much of the early work of the UN Office of Drugs and Crime (UNODC) and the Commission of Narcotics Drugs (CND) focused on restricting access to opioids and other controlled medicines as the primary means of reducing diversion.

It was the Cancer Control Unit of the World Health Organization (WHO), under the leadership of Jan Stjernswärd, that began to focus on palliative care and pain control as a global priority.[6] While a gradual increase in morphine consumption was seen in high-income countries, there was little increase in low- and middle-income countries.[7] The introduction of sustained-release formulations of morphine by pharmaceutical companies resulted in a further increase in consumption in those higher-income countries where it was marketed.

In the United States, increased utilization of morphine and other opioids was considered in response to increasing burden of untreated cancer pain. Based on the UK experience, in the 1980s the Wisconsin State Legislature asked the Wisconsin Controlled Substances Board to investigate the introduction of heroin for pain control in advanced cancer patients.[8] While the decision was made not to proceed with heroin, efforts were undertaken to pursue the use of morphine in the advanced cancer patient population. Early studies showed that even with increased licit morphine consumption in the state, there was no increase in diversion found throughout Wisconsin.[9] The Wisconsin Cancer Pain Initiative grew from these efforts of the Controlled Substances Board and faculty of the University of Wisconsin to focus on improving cancer pain relief, especially increased access to opioids in this appropriate medical indication.[10]

The World Health Organization included opioids, namely codeine and morphine, in its first Essential Medicines List.[11] WHO released a document promoting palliative care and addressing cancer pain relief with the introduction of the WHO three-step ladder.[12] Gradually opioid consumption increased in high-income countries such as those in North America, Europe, and Oceania, often with promotion by pharmaceutical companies. Currently most of the world's opioids are consumed by a small percentage of the world's population, leaving more than 80 percent with no access to pain relief. These are not just cancer patients but also patients dealing with obstetric needs, burns, trauma, and postoperative pain.

THE MEANING OF "CONTROLLED" ACCESS TO OPIOIDS

The reasons behind this maldistribution are multiple and have been documented by many, including the International Narcotic Control Board (INCB), the global body designated to control access to opioids. The use of the word "control" is suggested by many to mean "restrict," but the term is used as in "cancer control" or "quality control" or even "railway control."[13] The role of the board is to ensure that there is appropriate availability while also reducing the risk of diversion to nonmedical uses. The INCB has done multiple surveys of competent authorities (those responsible for opioid consumption in a country), which show that a diversity of barriers to access exists across the planet, but especially in noneconomically developed countries.[14] Some officials blame the INCB itself, while others blame fear of addiction or say that cost is a key component for lack of access.

ACHIEVING BALANCE

A balanced approach is needed to ensure that equitable access is achieved. The WHO has defined the principle of *balance* in opioid regulation,[15] confirmed in multiple UN resolutions, including the 2014 Palliative Care Resolution of the World Health Assembly and more recently the Vienna 2020 United Nations Commission on Narcotic Drugs:

> The Central Principle of "balance" represents a dual imperative of governments to establish a system of control to prevent abuse, trafficking, and diversion of narcotic drugs while, at the same time, ensuring their medical availability. While opioid analgesics are controlled drugs, they are also essential drugs and are absolutely necessary for the relief

of pain. Opioids, including those in the therapeutic group of morphine, should be accessible to all patients who need them for relief of pain. Governments must take steps to ensure the adequate availability of opioids for medical and scientific purposes. These steps include empowering medical practitioners to provide opioids in the course of professional practice, allowing them to prescribe, dispense and administer according to the individual medical needs of patients, and ensuring that a sufficient supply of opioids is available to meet medical demand.

When misused, opioids pose a threat to society; a system of control is necessary to prevent abuse, trafficking, and diversion, but the system of control is not intended to diminish the medical usefulness of opioids nor interfere in their legitimate medical uses and patient care. Indeed, governments have been asked to identify and remove impediments to the availability and medical use of opioid analgesics.

If governments are to "identify and remove impediments" to achieve a balanced approach to opioids, they must address three primary issues: medicine availability, appropriate policy, and education of clinicians, regulators, and patients. All three must be improved in concert. An advance of any one without the other two will not likely change the situation. For example, making oral morphine available in Ukraine without changing laws and policies together with educating physicians, nurses, pharmacists, patients, and even the police will not improve morphine's use in people such as Artur.

THE ROBIN HOOD OF UKRAINE

Artur died some three months after our visit, without needing to use his handgun. But the story of his ongoing care is enlightening. To ensure that he received more than the 50 mg of morphine allowed per day by Ukraine (and many other governments in the former Soviet Union), Artur was assisted by a modern-day Robin Hood. As other advanced cancer patients moved closer to the end of life and slipped into a coma, their families agreed to share morphine allocated for their family members with patients such as Artur. We were with him when he received one of these extra injections, and within twenty minutes of its administration, Artur was up and about both within the house and then the farmyard, checking on the dogs, chickens, and rabbits. In comparison to the gun he pulled from under his pillow, he pulled from a cage the largest rabbit I have ever seen. He was able to do so because of appropriate pain relief.

I was astounded by the actions of this "Robin Hood." I was filmed with him with the stated purpose of exploring the establishment of a hospice in this community, and this of course led to the need for better morphine availability for patients like Artur. I asked him about his methods, perhaps somewhat naïvely. To my surprise, he pulled out from deep within his satchel a small pouch, which he unrolled to produce a number of illegal morphine syringes, similar to the one he had given to Artur. Fear arose in my consciousness as I pondered the question, Is Robin Hood breaking the law? Are his actions legal? After further conversation through our interpreter, the answer came back. "No, it is not legal, and if we are caught it is punishable by three years in jail!"

My first thought was to wonder if it was better to be an Australian or an American in a Ukrainian prison. But as self-protection drifted from my mind, I asked myself the question, Would I be doing this in Australia or the United States, breaking the law in order to ensure my patients receive the pain relief required in the face of an advanced cancer diagnosis? The answer is clearly No!

Even to this day, I wrestle with my rationale for saying no. It is a fact that laws and regulations in the United States and most high-income countries allow the appropriate prescribing of opioids for cancer patients, but would I break the law if these hurdles were present in the United States? It is worth looking at the situation with opioid-related laws in the United States. While opioids were widely available in the 1920s, increasing concerns over their use led to prohibition, much as for alcohol. These restrictive US regulations persisted through to the 1970s, when, with the start of the modern hospice movement, awareness of the undertreatment of cancer pain grew.[16] Thankfully, regulations that had been a barrier to opioid prescriptions for cancer patients were loosened. But then the looser regulatory environment, coupled with overzealous marketing and poor, sometimes outright illegal, medical practice, resulted in a major increase in opioid consumption and associated deaths. A large percentage of these deaths were due to illicit or diverted opioids. The CDC promulgated tighter opioid regulations, leading to pain-management deficits in postoperative, chronic, and cancer pain management. This is despite the fact that the CDC guidelines were intended for primary care physicians and deliberately excluded cancer patients. Because of these regulations, I now have more issues with insurance companies approving the use of these medicines and pharmacies stocking them than concerns with federal and state laws over their use with cancer patients.[17]

So why am I not stretching these regulations for my US cancer patients who are struggling with access to pain medicines? My compliance with these regulations is, for one, a professional norm, but it is also associated with the greater good and the need to keep my license in order to manage the entire population of patients for whom I care. It is also important I keep my academic position for the ongoing education of colleagues and learners in the principles of palliative care. So, while not pushing me to illegal practice, Artur and his "Robin Hood" have strengthened my resolve to address the imbalance in access to opioids that exists throughout the world. All must work to create a system where narcotic restriction does not interfere with medical access to opioids. As the 1961 Single Convention on Narcotic Drugs stated, "The medical use of narcotic drugs [opioids] continues to be indispensable for the relief of pain and suffering . . . adequate provision must be made to ensure the availability of narcotic drugs [opioids] for such purposes." We must all work toward a time with the fierce urgency of now, when the Arturs and Vlads of the world do not consider suicide as a form of pain relief.

NOTES

1. Hastie et al. 2014; Cherny et al. 2013; Berterame et al. 2016; Knaul et al. 2018.
2. Cherny et al. 2010.
3. "NCD Mortality and Morbidity" n.d.
4. Saunders 1963.
5. Single Convention on Narcotic Drugs 1961, 1975, at 105.
6. Swerdlow and Stjernswärd 1982.
7. Cherny et al. 2010.
8. Dahl et al. 1988.
9. Joranson and Dahl 1989.
10. Dahl et al. 1988.
11. *Selection of Essential Drugs* 1977.
12. *Cancer Pain Relief* 1986.
13. Cleary, Husain, and Maurer 2016.
14. Berterame et al. 2016.
15. "Narcotic and Psychotropic Drugs" 2000; "Ensuring Balance in National Policies on Controlled Substances" 2011.
16. Dahl et al. 1988.
17. Cleary 2020.

WORKS CITED

Berterame, S., J. Erthal, J. Thomas, S. Fellner, B. Vosse, P. Clare, W. Hao, D. T. Johnson, A. Mohar, J. Pavadia, A. K. E. Samak, W. Sipp, V. Sumyai, S. Suryawati, J. Toufiq, R. Yans, and R. P. Mattick. 2016. "Use of and Barriers to Access to Opioid

Analgesics: A Worldwide, Regional, and National Study." *Lancet* 387 (10028): 1644–56.

Cherny, N. I., J. Baselga, F. de Conno, and L. Radbruch. 2010. "Formulary Availability and Regulatory Barriers to Accessibility of Opioids for Cancer Pain in Europe: A Report from the ESMO/EAPC Opioid Policy Initiative." *Annals of Oncology* 21 (3): 615–26.

Cherny, N. I., J. Cleary, W. Scholten, L. Radbruch, and J. Torode. 2013. "The Global Opioid Policy Initiative (GOPI) Project to Evaluate the Availability and Accessibility of Opioids for the Management of Cancer Pain in Africa, Asia, Latin America and the Caribbean, and the Middle East: Introduction and Methodology." *Annals of Oncology* 24 (Suppl 11): xi7–13.

Cleary, J. F. 2020. "Restoring Balance to Cancer Pain Management." *Cancer* 126 (4): 697–700.

Cleary, J. F., A. Husain, and M. Maurer. 2016. "Increasing Worldwide Access to Medical Opioids." *Lancet* 387 (10028): 1597–99.

Dahl, J. L., D. E. Joranson, D. Engber, and J. Dosch. 1988. "The Cancer Pain Problem: Wisconsin's Response." *Journal of Pain and Symptom Management* 3 (Suppl 3): S2–S20.

"Ensuring Balance in National Policies on Controlled Substances: Guidance for Availability and Accessibility of Controlled Medicines." 2011. World Health Organization. https://apps.who.int/iris/handle/10665/44519.

Hastie, B. A., A. M. Gilson, M. A. Maurer, and J. F. Cleary. 2014. "An Examination of Global and Regional Opioid Trends, 1980–2011." *Journal of Pain and Palliative Care Pharmacotherapy* 28 (3): 259–75.

Joranson, D. E., and J. L. Dahl. 1989. "An Analysis of Drug Use and Drug Diversion Following a Statewide Campaign for Improved Treatment of Severe Pain Due to Cancer: Report to

the US Public Health Service." Madison, WI.

Knaul, F. M., P. E. Farmer, E. L. Krakauer, L. De Lima, A. Bhadelia, X. Jiang Kwete, H. Arreola-Ornelas, O. Gómez-Dantés, N. M. Rodriguez, G. A. O. Alleyne, S. R. Connor, D. J. Hunter, D. Lohman, L. Radbruch, M. Del Rocío Sáenz Madrigal, R. Atun, K. M. Foley, J. Frenk, D. T. Jamison, M. R. Rajagopal, and Lancet Commission on Palliative Care and Pain Relief Study Group. 2018. "Alleviating the Access Abyss in Palliative Care and Pain Relief—An Imperative of Universal Health Coverage: The *Lancet* Commission Report." *Lancet* 391 (10128): 1391–454.

"Narcotic and Psychotropic Drugs: Achieving Balance in National Opioids Control Policy: Guidelines for Assessment." 2000. World Health Organization. https://apps.who.int/iris/handle/10665/66496.

"NCD Mortality and Morbidity." n.d. World Health Organization. Accessed September 11, 2020. https://www.who.int/gho/ncd/mortality_morbidity/en.

Saunders, C. 1963. "The Treatment of Intractable Pain in Terminal Cancer." *Proceedings of the Royal Society of Medicine* 56 (3): 195–97.

The Selection of Essential Drugs: Report of a WHO Expert Committee. 1977. World Health Organization Technical Report Series 615. Geneva: World Health Organization.

Single Convention on Narcotic Drugs, 1961, as Amended by the Protocol Amending the Single Convention on Narcotic Drugs, 1961. 1975. August 8, 1975. UNTS 976.

Swerdlow, M., and J. Stjernswärd. 1982. "Cancer Pain Relief—An Urgent Problem." *World Health Forum* 3:325–30.

World Health Organization. *Cancer Pain Relief*. 1986. Geneva: World Health Organization.

CHAPTER 11

Overcoming the Devastation Caused by Cultivated Ignorance About Pain and Opioid Addiction

Costantino Benedetti

The work that you are accomplishing is immensely important for the good of humanity, as you seek the ever more effective control of physical pain and the oppression of the mind and the spirit that physical pain often brings with it.

—POPE JOHN PAUL II, 1987

Anyone who has ever suffered severe pain knows the oppression of mind and spirit that such pain causes, and anyone who has ever suffered opioid addiction knows the same.[1] The twin scourges of inadequately treated pain and opioid addiction derive from our collective ignorance of the science and practice of treating both severe pain (acute or chronic) and opioid addiction. In this essay, I will share my personal analysis based upon my five decades in pain therapy and palliative medicine, hoping to shine light on the darkness, starting with the inadequate education of medical professionals and public policy–makers regarding pain management and the impact this had on the opioid epidemic. Following the historical journey through both problems, I will offer the reader a prescription for the future of pain management.

THE MAGNITUDE OF THE PROBLEMS

In 2011, the Institute of Medicine (IOM) reported that over 100 million Americans suffered from chronic pain.[2] This number included people whose pain ranged from mild, with little effect on activities of daily living, to "high-impact pain" so severe it prevented the individual from engaging in most basic physical and psychosocial activities. Such high-impact pain is experienced by approximately twenty-five million adult Americans.[3] Opioid addiction, experienced by over two million Americans,[4] not only destroys livelihoods and families but destroys life—it kills. Forty-nine thousand deaths were attributed to opioid overdose in 2018.[5] High-impact pain also destroys lives and families, but we have no hard data on resulting mortality associated with high-impact pain, for pain is not a reportable cause of death. That does not mean it is not sometimes a cause of death, for, at a minimum, among the deleterious effects of poorly treated pain is an increased risk of suicide.[6]

The same 2011 IOM report noted that over 40 percent of all physician visits are prompted by pain complaints, yet American medical students received only nine to eleven hours of pain education over four years. Not surprising given the lack of education, 68 percent of all academic primary care physicians felt unprepared to treat chronic pain.[7] With that level of faculty discomfort managing chronic pain, it is not surprising that medical trainees are not provided adequate education on the topic.

Poorly treated high-impact pain, opioid addiction, and inadequate medical training in these arenas should leave no doubt in anyone's mind about the seriousness of the problem we face. A reasonably efficacious approach to facing this problem will require the accomplishment of three tasks:

1. Better dissemination of the past hundred years of basic science and clinical pain research
2. Ongoing acquisition and dissemination of newer basic science and clinical pain research
3. Reversal of misconceptions surrounding chronic pain and opioid addiction

A BRIEF HISTORY OF PAIN THERAPY

Modern pain management began with the work of Dr. George Washington Crile, a surgeon and one of the founders of the Cleveland Clinic. Dr. Crile and his colleague Dr. William Lower published a small book in 1914 entitled

Anoci-Association, which means "without the association of nociception."[8] They articulated three essential principles of pain therapy:

1. Severe pain has serious deleterious effects—even death—and must be taken seriously.
2. Pain should be considered a neurologic disease.
3. Pain therapy must be individualized.

Severe Pain Can Kill

The first major principle described by Dr. Crile was that severe pain could have serious physical effects on the body, including the demise of the patient. He noted that in 1908 the mortality rate associated with surgery performed at his hospital in Cleveland was 4.4 percent. Dr. Crile instituted better management of perioperative anxiety and postoperative pain, and by 1912 the mortality rate had dropped to 1.9 percent (fig. 11.1). Contemporary physicians will hypothesize that many variables might have improved perioperative mortality, but the main explanation, Dr. Crile believed, was improved pain control. A more recent study meeting more modern research standards and coming to the same conclusion will be described later.

MORTALITY RATE

MORTALITY RATE	1	2	3	4	5	6	7
1908							
1912							
1913							

FIG. 11.1 Comparison of the mortality rate of all operations performed at Lakeside Hospital by George W. Crile and William E. Lower and their resident staff during 1908—the year before anoci-association was introduced—with the mortality rate of 1912 and 1913. G. W. Crile and W. E. Lower, *Anoci-Association*, ed. Amy F. Rowland (Philadelphia: W. B. Saunders, 1914), 221.

Pain Should Be Considered a Neurologic Disease

The second major principle proposed by Dr. Crile was that pain, especially chronic pain, was caused by changes in the nervous system, making pain a neurologic disease. Crile and Lower wrote, "Pain is not at the site of the incision but in a part of the brain. . . . A strong traumatic or psychic stimulus produces some changes in the conductivities somewhere in its cerebral arc, the effect of which is to lower the threshold of that arc . . . and hence from that time on, mere trifles become adequate stimuli." While this early characterization of the aberrant responses to stimuli is not entirely accurate (pain may be localized to the actual site of injury, such as a neuroma within scar tissue), they correctly recognized that a strong emotional stimulus may have long-term effects on pain perception. Under normal conditions, the nervous system responds to high-intensity mechanical, chemical, or thermal stimuli, leading to the conscious perception of pain. But strong pain also activates the limbic system and the frontal lobe of the brain, triggering the emotional responses associated with the perception of pain. Emotional status can either facilitate or hinder the transmission of nociceptive pain impulses. In addition, the nervous system, once activated by nociception, may develop changes to the somatosensory cortex leading to abnormal perceptions of pain, including hyperalgesia (an exaggerated perception of pain caused by a painful stimulus) and allodynia (a perception of pain caused by a stimulus that is nonpainful under normal conditions). Both phenomena support the importance of recognizing pain as a neurologic disorder.[9]

The Personalization of Pain Therapy

The third principle described by Dr. Crile was that pain therapy must be individualized and titrated to analgesic effect. It would be another four decades before science and medical practice caught up with this groundbreaking assertion. In the 1950s, Lasagna and Beecher noted that 10 mg of intramuscular morphine (the standard dose at the time) controlled the pain of only 65 percent of surgical postoperative patients.[10] A standard dose of morphine was clearly inadequate pain control for many patients. Individualized dose adjustment was needed, just as Dr. Crile had advocated. The concept was even more clearly demonstrated by Dodson in 1982, when she performed a simple study that should be known to every health-care professional treating patients with pain.[11] The study involved forty-nine patients receiving morphine analgesia after surgery using a patient-controlled analgesia (PCA) device. To better illustrate the results, the data reported by Dodson are displayed in table 11.1.

TABLE 11.1   Doses of self-administered morphine used by forty-nine patients to control postoperative pain using patient-controlled analgesia

mg/h of morphine	Number of patients	Percentage of patients
0–0.5	2	4.1%
0.6–1.0	3	6.1%
1.1–1.5	8	16.3%
1.6–2.0	7	14.3%
2.1–2.5	12	24.5%
2.6–3.0	6	12.2%
3.1–3.5	4	8.2%
3.6–4.0	3	6.1%
4.1–4.5	2	4.1%
4.6–5.0	0	0.0%
5.1–5.5	1	2.0%
5.6–8.5	0	0.0%
8.6–9.0	1	2.0%

Two patients used less than or equal to 0.5 mg of morphine every hour, while one patient at the other extreme used between 8.6 and 9 mg of morphine every hour. It is clear that if every patient had received the same amount of morphine, the great majority of patients would have been either undertreated or overtreated by the analgesic. Additionally, it is revealing that the data from Dodson are very similar to the data from Lasagna and Beecher thirty years earlier. In the Lasagna and Beecher study, 10 mg of injectable morphine provided analgesia after surgery for only 65 percent of the patients. In Dodson's study, 64.7 percent of patients were able to control their pain by using 2.5 mg or less of morphine per hour (10 mg or less every four hours), showing that the two studies are consistent with one another.

Variability in response to opioids was further confirmed through basic science research demonstrating that in a rodent model, weak responders to opioid-induced pain relief needed up to one hundred times the dose of morphine as strong responders.[12]

FROM PAST TO PRESENT: THE EVOLUTION OF PAIN MEDICINE

To better understand the present state of pain medicine, a further review of its evolution following Drs. Crile and Lower's work is useful. Their insights were developed at a time when research was spotty and not up to contemporary standards and the dissemination of new ideas was challenging. The three principles of pain management postulated were not widely accepted by the medical community of their day. Such acceptance would have to wait several decades until 1944 and the Second World War, when Dr. John Bonica, a twenty-seven-year-old recent anesthesiology graduate, was appointed director of anesthesia at the Madigan Army Hospital. His duties included managing pain associated with the wounds of injured soldiers. He recalled that he had never received education on pain medicine and asked his colleagues from different subspecialties, including surgery, internal medicine, orthopedics, and neurology, to help in this endeavor. They all admitted to having very limited knowledge related to pain management.[13] Bonica found that the best, albeit limited, way of treating the most difficult pain patients was to involve specialists of varied disciplines. He hypothesized that face-to-face open discussion across disciplines would significantly improve diagnosis and treatment of pain, thus creating the first multidisciplinary approach to pain management.

Nine years after being assigned this pain-management duty, he published the first comprehensive textbook on pain therapy, *The Management of Pain*.[14] Among other insights, and much like Dr. Crile thirty years prior, he noted an association between improved analgesia and decreased mortality, suggesting that the difference could be attributed to three significant pathologic effects of acute pain, which he described as reflexes.

The first reflex was the muscular spasm and vasoconstriction associated with severe acute pain. Muscular spasm can be beneficial when it immobilizes a fractured long bone like a femur, preventing further injury, and vasoconstriction can prevent exsanguination from a torn artery. However, these same reflexes, when associated with severe pain in the upper abdomen or thorax (intended via surgery or unintended via accident or illness), decrease the patient's ability to breathe, lower functional residual capacity (FRC), and cause hypoventilation, hypoxemia (low oxygen), hypercarbia (high carbon dioxide), respiratory acidosis, atelectasis, pneumonia, and eventually respiratory failure.[15] While hypoxemia may be corrected with supplemental oxygen, treatment of hypercarbia and respiratory acidosis requires either resolution of the pain-induced muscular spasm or intubation and mechanical ventilation. This "reflex" is even more dangerous in patients with underlying pulmonary conditions (e.g., COPD), and it may be instigated by nontraumatic conditions causing pain. I have personally treated a case of thoracic herpes zoster–related pain resulting in muscular spasm–associated hypoventilation.

By careful titration of opioids, pain relief was achieved, normal ventilation was restored, and respiratory depression requiring intubation was prevented. As for the deleterious consequences of postoperative thoracic pain, the former director of thoracic surgery at the Ohio State University James Cancer Hospital would not start a surgery until a functional thoracic epidural catheter was placed to provide continuous postoperative epidural analgesia.

The second "reflex" noted by Dr. Bonica was that severe pain caused the release of cortisol and catecholamines. Cortisol decreases the immune response, potentially contributing to infection, while catecholamines increase heart rate, peripheral vascular resistance, and blood pressure. This in turn increases cardiac work and oxygen demand, which in the setting of coronary artery disease may lead to angina, myocardial infarction, heart failure, and even death! This sequence of events is well known in the postanesthesia care unit (PACU), where it is abundantly clear that severe postoperative pain must be corrected to prevent this potentially catastrophic cascade of events.

Finally, Bonica's third "reflex" described the phenomenon of severe, poorly treated pain resulting in neurologically mediated emotional responses including fear, anxiety, and voluntary immobility. Immobility, the simple failure to move, leads to weakness and deconditioning and increases the risk of deep vein thrombosis and potentially fatal pulmonary embolism. This reflex underscores the importance of acute pain control.

Responding to the evidence that severe, poorly treated pain was associated with increased morbidity and mortality, a service totally dedicated to the treatment of acute pain was developed in 1985 at the University of Washington, becoming the blueprint for modern hospital acute pain services.[16] In 1987, a seminal study found that high-risk elderly surgical patients with significant heart or lung disease had fewer postoperative complications when optimal pain control with continuous intraspinal analgesia was provided rather than standard intravenous analgesia.[17] After giving informed consent to the study, the patients were randomized in two groups: one of continuous epidural analgesia (Group I) and one of the hospital standard pain control through IV analgesia (Group II). It should be noted that administration of epidural analgesia has been proven to provide significantly stronger pain relief than IV administration. The results were as follows for Group I versus Group II: mortality 0 percent versus 16 percent; cardiovascular failure 14.3 percent versus 52 percent; respiratory failure 10.7 percent versus 32 percent; major infection 7.1 percent versus 40 percent; average ICU days 2.5 versus 5.7;

hours of mechanical ventilation 7.1 versus 81.8. The average cost per patient for Group I was $14,109, while the average cost per patient for Group II was $25,541. It should be noted that I did not adjust these costs for inflation, and that medical costs are now significantly higher. The study was supposed to include one hundred patients, but for ethical reasons, due to the drastic difference in results, it was stopped at fifty-three patients (Group I had twenty-eight and Group II had twenty-five). Due to the number of patients studied, the difference in mortality rate did not reach statistical significance. All the other parameters were significantly different, with the epidural group having better outcomes across multiple parameters compared to the standard analgesia therapy group and lower cost. Therefore, effective postoperative pain control should be provided not only for the humanitarian reason of decreasing suffering but also for a positive economic effect to the hospital. This study adds further credence to Dr. Crile's 1914 assertion that inadequately treated postoperative pain causes increased mortality, especially in high-risk surgical patients.

These clinical findings and interventions were accompanied by a growing body of basic science research into the pathophysiology of pain. In a series of studies from 1980 to 1994, John Liebeskind and associates at the University of California Los Angeles studied the effects of inescapable (chronic) pain and acute postoperative pain in animals. They found that both caused a significant depression of the immune system—in particular, a decrease in the number of natural killer cells, which are thought to play a role in the prevention of cancer. In these experiments, rats were either exposed to inescapable pain, acute pain, or no pain at all (control group). All were then injected with the same type and number of cancer cells. Cancer developed in a significantly higher number of the animals exposed to either type of pain compared to the control group.[18] We do not know if this same phenomenon occurs in humans, but it is of interest that at least three studies have suggested improved survival in metastatic cancer patients who receive early palliative care referral, and some have speculated that this improved survival could be related to better pain control.[19]

Pain Medicine and the Birth of Palliative Medicine

In 1953, Dr. Bonica foretold the need for palliative medicine when commenting on organized medicine's failure to adequately manage cancer pain and associated suffering, writing: "The deplorable attitude of defeatism and apathetic therapeutic inactivity [toward pain control] . . . must be abandoned and replaced by courageous aggressiveness tempered by sane judgement." He suggested multiple interventions, such as "psychological support" and "the sympathy, the understanding, the kindness, [and] the moral support of their physician." He continued, "It is an alleviation of misery not to suffer alone," and emphasized that "supportive measures are also necessary," such as "nourishing food, good hygiene, and competent nursing care." Palliative medicine professionals will surely recognize in Dr. Bonica's 1953 insights many of the building blocks of palliative medicine.

In 1967, Dr. Cicely Saunders opened St. Christopher's Hospice in London, starting the modern hospice movement, promoting the relief of physical pain as a fundamental goal. In 1973, after visiting St. Christopher's Hospice, Dr. Balfour Mount of McGill University started the palliative care movement in Canada. Many other pioneers in palliative medicine passed through St. Christopher's, including one of the other authors of this book, Dr. Declan Walsh, founder of the first palliative care program in the United States.

Dr. Bonica was not only a physician researcher; he was an organizer. In 1973, he invited over three hundred international specialists for a week-long meeting in a converted, isolated convent in Issaquah, Washington. This setting allowed for formal presentations and informal discussions. The founding of the International Association for the Study of Pain (IASP) and the establishment of the *Journal of Pain* under the leadership of Dr. Patrick Wall both grew out of this meeting.

This was followed by the first International World Meeting on Advanced Cancer Pain in Venice, Italy, in 1978. Following this meeting, the director of the World Health Organization (WHO) Cancer Pain Program asked Dr. Bonica to lead the development of a basic guideline for the treatment of cancer pain.

This led to the stepladder approach to pain management, adjusting therapy based on pain intensity and functional impairment. As important as this guideline was, there were problems. For example, codeine, a weak opioid analgesic associated with significantly more side effects than morphine, including more nausea, vomiting, and severe constipation, was included, dictated by the reality that in many nations of the world codeine was and is the only opioid available. In addition, even though the guidelines were translated, published, and distributed in many different countries, formal pain medicine education remained minimal.

By the 1980s, the pioneers of pain medicine and patient advocacy groups sought to inform society at large—not just the medical community—that pain could and must be effectively treated. They reached out to the public via print media (newspapers and periodicals like *Time* and *People* magazines) and television interviews. In 1990, Dr. Ron Melzack published a seminal article in *Scientific American* entitled "The Tragedy of Needless Pain," conveying to the public that poorly treated pain was common yet better pain control was possible.[20]

Unfortunately, most physicians continued to have limited knowledge of pain medicine and struggled to treat severe pain in conditions like cancer. I believe that this failure to meet the challenge of uncontrolled pain became a driver of the physician-assisted suicide movement. This movement led Pope John Paul II in the encyclical *Evangelium vitae* (1995) to write that euthanasia was not a solution to intractable pain, but palliative care was. Two years later the Supreme Court of the United States declared that neither physician-assisted suicide nor active euthanasia was constitutionally protected, but effective palliative care was (*Washington v. Glucksberg*, 521 US 702 [1997]).

Medical Education Deficits in Pain Medicine

As more knowledge accumulated about pain assessment and management, the call for increased education of health care professionals continued. As previously cited, in 2010 only 32 percent of academic primary care physicians felt qualified to treat (and presumably to teach the management of) pain.[21]

The late Professor Ben Rich, a lawyer, judge, and ethicist, wrote extensively about the failure of academic medicine to teach pain assessment, management, and opioid pharmacology, ultimately leading to our contemporary opioid crisis—the excessive treatment of mild and short-lived pain, the undertreatment of severe cancer pain, the mistreatment of chronic pain, and the furtherance of opioid addiction. He observed that the "consistent failure of the medical profession to address these deficits in the education of physicians renders it vulnerable to the charge that it has actually cultivated its ignorance about the assessment and management of pain and the integral relationship between pain relief and acceptable patient care."[22]

Cultivated ignorance may well have contributed to the misprescribing and abuse of Oxycontin. In the late 1990s, the manufacturer of Oxycontin launched a marketing campaign aimed at convincing primary care physicians to prescribe their product. Oxycontin's manufacturer claimed the new product was more easily administered as it was long-acting, similar to already available long-acting morphine used primarily for cancer pain, providing twelve hours of analgesia when the most commonly used opioids of the time worked for only about four hours. In reality, the analgesic effect of Oxycontin lasted only eight hours in many patients. The company then suggested a variety of strategies for bridging the four-hour gap, including using more short-acting oxycodone or increasing the dose of Oxycontin to prolong its duration of action, both of which reasonably contributed to higher overall opioid consumption and probably addiction. But why was the pharmaceutical industry able to mislead an incredible number of physicians in the improper prescribing of Oxycontin? I believe lack of professional education, as outlined above, was a major contributor.

Pain, particularly severe pain, is a subjective and emotional experience, which makes it one of the most challenging conditions for physicians to assess and treat. Ideally, the more challenging the condition, the more medical education required. In medical conditions not associated with subjective experience (blood pressure, for example), medication misuse usually manifests as underuse, taking less medication than prescribed. Because a patient subjectively feels the pain return as a medication wears off (generally not the case in an example such as blood pressure), pain medication misuse more often manifests as additional doses taken more often than prescribed. Most physicians overestimate the duration of action of any specific opioid. Consequently, patients may seem to be misusing medication by taking more than prescribed in order to achieve adequate relief (pseudoaddiction).

At this point it is very important to define addiction, misuse, and abuse, as these terms are often used inappropriately. Addiction is defined as a behavioral disorder involving craving of the drug for reasons other than pain control and compulsive attempts to obtain the drug despite harm. Therefore, tolerance and physical dependence are necessary but not sufficient signs of addiction. Misuse occurs when a patient uses a prescribed medication for the appropriate indication but not in the prescribed fashion. Historically, the use of a medication for a condition other than the original condition for which the medication was prescribed has been referred to as "abuse." For consistency with the studies cited here, and because this chapter provides a historical perspective, I will continue to use this definition. However, it must be acknowledged that the term "abuse" has a derogatory connotation, and that at the time of writing, medical researchers and practitioners are making a concerted effort to eliminate this and other stigmatizing language. As an alternative, researchers are simply using the phrase "used other than prescribed."

A clinical example will help illustrate the concepts of misuse and abuse. A patient with severe pain caused by metastatic prostate cancer is prescribed 15 mg of oxycodone for pain. The patient is told to take it every six hours, but severe pain begins to return after four hours. The patient asks the oncologist for enough medication to take it every four hours, but this is denied. The patient is now in a no-win situation. Follow the physician's advice and live with two hours of uncontrolled pain out of every six hours, or "misuse" the medication, taking it every four hours and running out of the medicine early. The oncologist may even believe the patient is addicted, when in fact the patient displays "pseudo-addiction," appearing addicted only because the physician is unfamiliar with opioid pharmacology. If the same patient has difficulty sleeping at night due to anxiety about what will happen to his family after his death and takes oxycodone to sleep, he is engaged in abuse of the oxycodone as the drug is not prescribed nor appropriate for treatment of anxiety or insomnia. Ideally, the oncologist would have better knowledge of the analgesic duration of oxycodone and might also recognize anxiety as a cause of sleep disturbance, treating both circumstances appropriately. However, a supportive palliative care referral could be even more helpful, as palliative care specialists and their teammates are better able to address what Cicely Saunders described as "total pain," the physical, emotional, spiritual, and social distress experienced by patients with serious and life-threatening diseases.[23]

The Opioid Crisis: From Pain Science to Flawed Public Policy

As the scientific and clinical medicine knowledge base of pioneering pain management specialists was translated into public education and policy, chronic pain became labeled a public health problem. The concept of "Pain as the Fifth Vital Sign" was introduced in the United States to deal with this problem by the Joint Commission for the Accreditation of Health Care Organizations. For each patient encounter, in addition to obtaining the four classic vital signs (heart rate, respiratory rate, temperature, and blood pressure), the patient was also asked to rate his or her pain on a scale of 0–10 (0 being no pain and 10 being the worst possible, unbearable, and excruciating pain). Unfortunately, while the idea of routine pain assessment was reasonable, it was poorly implemented by physicians and nurses who were inadequately educated about pain. For example, providers were told that all pain scores of 5 or more required an intervention, which many presumed meant providing more pain medication, instead of taking the additional step to assess the impact of pain on the patient. This practice failed to incorporate Dr. Crile's 1914 recommendation for individualized pain therapy, Lasagna and Beecher's 1954 observations on optimal morphine dosing, and Dodson's 1982 demonstration of individual variability in opioid needs to treat pain.

Pain is a subjective experience and different for every patient. A pain level that is tolerable for one person may be intolerable for another. Adding a simple inquiry into the patient's tolerance of their pain level can obviate the need for additional opioids in many cases. Physicians inadequately trained in pain management also fail to take into account the likely duration of need, prescribing many weeks' worth of opioids for acute, short-lived problems like a dental extraction or a sprained ankle, which may often be adequately treated with other analgesics such as a combination of acetaminophen and nonsteroidal anti-inflammatory drugs. However, if the latter combination fails to provide tolerable pain relief, short-term opioids may then be prescribed. Still other physicians overprescribed opioids out of fear they would be penalized for inadequate treatment of the new fifth vital sign. The net result of overprescription born from ignorance and perverse incentives was an ever-increasing supply of opioids available for both abuse and diversion for illegal use.[24]

Opioid Addiction in the Twenty-First Century

Opioid addiction is often described as an overwhelming problem in the United States. Although this statement is true, I am concerned that frequently cited statistics about the magnitude of the problem and the addictiveness of opioids are often presented in a misleading fashion, a practice that contributes to the cultivated ignorance described in this chapter. For example, to emphasize the scope of the problem it has been stated that 99 percent of the hydrocodone used in the world is consumed in the United States. True, but hydrocodone is not sold in most other countries, nor do most countries collect national data on opioid prescriptions.

It is also routinely stated that opioids are highly addictive, and at first glance this might seem incontrovertible. After all, statistics from the Center for Behavioral Health Statistics and Quality tell us that about two million Americans are addicted to opioids.[25] Although this number is surely unacceptable, estimates from the National Survey of Drug Use and Health (NSDUH) show that in 2015, 37.8 percent of civilian noninstitutionalized US adults (approximately 91.8 million) used opioids at least once in the last twelve months.[26] In this study, although addiction is not reported on specifically, only 2.1 percent of those who used opioids in the last twelve months reported disordered use, suggesting that the vast majority of those who use opioids do not experience addiction or other forms of disordered use. In addition, there are unconfirmed reports of individuals becoming addicted to opioids after only a few exposures. Although I have not observed this personally, in light of the heterogeneity of opioid pharmacogenetics, it is conceivable that a small number of individuals could experience this. However, even among chronic pain patients taking opioids on a daily basis for months or even years, opioid addiction is relatively low. The NIH has reported that among individuals treated for chronic pain, 14–19 percent of chronic opioid users are addicted, depending upon the definition of addiction applied.[27] Stated another way, even among chronic pain patients, the majority do not become addicted.

Although opioids may be less addictive than widely believed, one cannot simply ignore the reality of two million addicts. In 2010, the Centers for Disease Control and Prevention (CDC) reported that since the 1990s there had been a 300 percent increase in opioid prescriptions and a similar increase in opioid-associated deaths, all attributed to overdose.[28] No wonder both the CDC and Drug Enforcement Administration (DEA) sought to decrease opioid addiction. But how accurate was their analysis, and how appropriate was their approach to the challenge?

Might additional factors beyond overprescribing have also contributed to the obvious rise of opioid misuse and deaths attributed to opioid addiction? Several million citizens suffered the despair of job loss during the great recession of 2007–8. The relationship between job loss and opioid abuse has not been adequately studied, but I believe it is reasonable to speculate some relationship. In addition, it may not be accurate to label all overdose deaths as "accidental." Anecdotal reports from several persons who survived an opiate overdose revealed an intentionality and even hope that their last injection would be fatal. The 2010 CDC report did not distinguish between patients with legitimate versus illegitimate opioid use, nor did it place deaths due to opioids within the context of other drug-related deaths. For example, in the late 1990s, Singh reported 107,000 hospitalizations and 16,500 deaths annually attributable to prescription nonsteroidal anti-inflammatory drug use, more than the 14,800 reported annually attributable to opioid use.[29]

Following their analysis of the problem, the CDC developed guidelines for chronic pain therapy.[30] The guidelines focused on the lack of evidence to demonstrate the efficacy of opioid use for the treatment of chronic pain and emphasized the harm that can result from chronic opioid use. The guidelines recommended caution when using morphine milligram equivalents (MME) greater than 50 MME/day. Several prominent organizations, including the American Cancer Society, the American Medical Association, and the American Academy of Pain Medicine, openly decried these guidelines, anticipating the harm such a restrictive approach could have on patients already managing their pain with prescription opioids, and the impact on future pain patients.[31]

The efforts of the CDC to curtail the use of prescription opioids had a chilling effect on physicians, especially primary care providers, who either stopped prescribing opioids, decreased the amount drastically, or stopped treating patients with chronic pain. Several years of physician implementation of the CDC recommendations have resulted in significant harm to a large number of chronic pain patients.[32] Although opioid prescriptions decreased about 25 percent (as intended), deaths associated with both the licit and illicit opioid overdose increased over 300 percent (from 14,800 in 2010 to 47,600 in 2017), and the trend continues to be unfavorable.[33] These numbers also fail to include deaths attributable to complications of illicit drug use, including the use of contaminated needles, which can lead to blood-borne diseases such as HIV, hepatitis C, and serious bacterial infections.

There are likely several reasons for this paradoxical outcome. The drop in licit opioids was associated with an increase in illicit opioids, the latter associated with unpredictable opioid products, which may result in unintentional overdose. Another potential contributor to overdose deaths may have been the replacement of opioid drug-maintenance programs with total abstinence programs. In an abstinence program, the patient is withdrawn completely from opioids, usually during one month of inpatient therapy, resulting in a loss of tolerance to opioids. If the patient later relapses and takes an opioid dose that might have been tolerated when actively addicted, that previously tolerated opioid dose may prove to be a lethal overdose when tolerance has been lost.

It should be noted that in the last few years, the recommended treatment for opioid addiction has included a longitudinal multimodal treatment approach. This includes psychosocial interventions and pharmacological treatment of addiction consisting of methadone or, preferably, suboxone.

The United States is not the only country to have a problem with opioid addiction. In the early 2000s, Portugal was in the midst of a significant drug abuse crisis. In contrast to the criminalization and abstinence approach of the United States, Portugal implemented a chronic opioid maintenance program for opioid addiction, treating it as a medical problem rather than a moral failure or crime. By 2016, the mortality rate for drug overdose in Portugal was 6 per 1,000,000 inhabitants, while in the United States it was 186 per 1,000,000.[34]

The unintended deleterious effects of the CDC chronic pain management guidelines were not surprising to many pain-management specialists, but they were real nonetheless. In 2019, the lead author of the guidelines reported in the *New England Journal of Medicine* that their recommendations had been misinterpreted by physicians, resulting in harm caused to patients with chronic pain.[35] That same year, the department of Health and Human Services (HHS) released revised guidelines.[36] The main tenets of chronic pain treatment put forth by the new guidelines required close collaboration between the physician and patient in assessing the need to taper opioids and the speed at which to do it. They also emphasized that some patients with chronic pain will need long-term opioid treatment.[37]

CONCLUSION: A PRESCRIPTION FOR THE FUTURE

It is encouraging that restrictions on legitimate opioid use are beginning to change, especially for patients with chronic pain. In the 2019 *New England Journal of Medicine* perspective essay "No Shortcuts to Safer Opioid Prescribing," Dowell (a CDC physician) and colleagues recognized that the CDC guidelines had caused unintended patient harm and offered many wise suggestions for the future.[38] However, as positive as these refinements might be, I believe that the path to overcoming the twin scourges of undertreatment of pain and opioid addiction will require dedicated research and, even more importantly, better education. Future research could even include treatments yet to be discovered that are as or more effective and safer than opioids. The "cultivated ignorance" of my profession must come to an end. Medical school faculty involved in the active care of patients must be prepared to manage acute and chronic pain and to teach pain management and opioid pharmacology to their students. The teaching must start with the basic sciences, then move into the anatomy, physiology, and psychology of pain, the pharmacology of opioids and other agents, and ultimately the clinical practice of pain management, not only by pain management or palliative medicine experts but by all physicians who care for patients with painful conditions. The principles of pain management first outlined by Dr. Crile and further validated and refined by Drs. Lasagna, Beecher, Bonica, Dodson, and others must be taken to heart. Only then can we obtain the balance needed to manage the twin scourges faced by our patients, the healing professions, and our society.

NOTES

I would like to thank my daughter, Dr. Giulia Benedetti, who transcribed this chapter with me and contributed to the editing process. For further discussion on this topic, a recorded lecture entitled "Advocacy for the Ever More Effective Control of Physical Pain" is publicly available on YouTube (https://www.youtube.com/watch?v=YZlmSPDpLy4).

1. Epigraph: John Paul II 1987. See also Benedetti, Chapman, and Giron 1990, xiii–xiv.
2. Institute of Medicine (US) Committee on Advancing Pain Research, Care, and Education 2011.
3. Dahlhamer et al. 2018.
4. Center for Behavioral Health Statistics and Quality 2016.
5. Scholl et al. 2019.
6. Petrosky et al. 2018.
7. Institute of Medicine (US) Committee on Advancing Pain Research, Care, and Education 2011, 196.
8. Crile and Lower 1914.
9. Cervero 2009; Morpurgo and Spinelli 1976.
10. Lasagna and Beecher 1954.
11. Dodson 1982.
12. Panocka, Marek, and Sadowski 1986.
13. Benedetti 1987.
14. Bonica 1953, 1422–25.
15. Benedetti and Premuda 1990.
16. Ready et al. 1988.
17. Yeager et al. 1987.
18. Page et al. 1993.
19. Temel et al. 2010; Bakitas et al. 2014; Sullivan et al. 2019.
20. Melzack 1990.
21. Institute of Medicine (US) Committee on Advancing Pain Research, Care, and Education 2011.
22. Rich 2006.
23. Richmond 2005.
24. Wee Jun Yan, Lim Tian Ying, and Brennan 2018.
25. Center for Behavioral Health Statistics and Quality 2016.
26. Han et al. 2017.
27. National Institutes of Health 2014.
28. National Center for Injury Prevention and Control and Division of Unintentional Injury Prevention 2011.
29. Singh 1998.
30. Dowell, Haegerich, and Chou 2016.
31. Rose 2018.
32. Dowell, Haegerich, and Chou 2019.
33. Scholl et al. 2019.
34. Perry 2017.
35. Dowell, Haegerich, and Chou 2019.
36. US Department of Health and Human Services Working Group 2019.
37. Dowell, Compton, and Giroir 2019.
38. Dowell, Haegerich, and Chou 2019.

WORKS CITED

Bakitas, M., T. Tosteson, Z. Li, K. Lyons, J. Hull, Z. Li, J. N. Dionne-Odom, J. Frost, M. Hegel, A. Azuero, T. Ahles, J. R. Rigas, J. M. Pipas, and K. H. Dragnev. 2014. "The ENABLE III Randomized Controlled Trial of Concurrent Palliative Oncology Care." *Journal of Clinical Oncology* 32 (15 Suppl): 9512.

Benedetti, C. 1987. "Wrestling with Pain: John J. Bonica, MD. Autobiography." Lecture given July 1987 at the International Symposium on Opioid Analgesia Honoring His Seventieth Birthday. Video posted March 14, 2017. https://www.youtube.com/watch?v=IQ_lJby_owM.

Benedetti, C., C. R. Chapman, and G. Giron, eds. 1990. *Opioid Analgesia: Recent Advances in Systemic Administration. Advances in Pain Research and Therapy* 14. New York: Raven Press.

Benedetti, C., E. D. Dickerson, and L. L. Nichols. 2001. "Medical Education: A Barrier to Pain Therapy and Palliative Care." *Journal of Pain and Symptom Management* 21 (5): 360–62.

Benedetti, C., and L. Premuda. 1990. "The History of Opium and Its Derivatives." In Benedetti, Chapman, and Giron, *Opioid Analgesia*, 1–35.

Bonica, J. 1953. *The Management of Pain.* Philadelphia: Lippincott, Williams, and Wilkins.

Carli, F. 2014. "Henrik Kehlet, M.D., Ph.D., Recipient of the 2014 Excellence in Research Award." *Anesthesiology* 121 (4): 690–91.

Center for Behavioral Health Statistics and Quality. 2016. "Key Substance Use and Mental Health Indicators in the United States: Results from the 2015 National Survey on Drug Use and Health." HHS Publication No. SMA 16-4984, NSDUH Series H-51. https://www.samhsa.gov/data/sites/default/files/NSDUH-FFR1-2015Rev/NSDUH-FFR1-2015Rev/NSDUH-FFR1-2015Rev/NSDUH-National%20Findings-REVISED-2015.pdf.

Cervero, F. 2009. "Pain: Friend or Foe? A Neurologic Perspective: The 2008 Bonica Aware Lecture." *Regional Anesthesia and Pain Medicine* 34 (6): 569–74.

Crile, G. W., and W. E. Lower. 1914. *Anoci-Association.* Edited by A. F. Rowland. Philadelphia: W. B. Saunders.

Dahlhamer, J., J. Lucas, C. Zelaya, R. Nahin, S. Mackey, L. DeBar, R. Kerns, M. Von Korff, L. Porter, and C. Helmick. 2018. "Prevalence of Chronic Pain and High-Impact Chronic Pain Among Adults—United States, 2016." *Morbidity and Mortality Weekly Report* 67 (36): 1001–6.

Dodson, M. E. 1982. "A Review of Methods for Relief of Postoperative Pain." *Annals of the Royal College of Surgeons of England* 64 (5): 324–27.

Dowell, D., W. M. Compton, and B. P. Giroir. 2019. "Patient-Centered Reduction or Discontinuation of Long-Term Opioid Analgesics: The HHS Guide for Clinicians." *JAMA* 322 (19): 1855–56.

Dowell, D., T. M. Haegerich, and R. Chou. 2016. "CDC Guideline for Prescribing Opioids for Chronic Pain—United States, 2016." *Morbidity and Mortality Weekly Report Recommendations and Reports* 65 (1): 1–49.

———. 2019. "No Shortcuts to Safer Opioid Prescribing." *New England Journal of Medicine* 380 (24): 2285–87.

Fishman, S. M. 2006. "Commentary in Response to Paulozzi et al.: Prescription Drug Abuse and Safe Pain Management." *Pharmacoepidemiology and Drug Safety* 15 (9): 628–31.

Han, B., W. M. Compton, C. Blanco, E. Crane, J. Lee, and C. M. Jones. 2017. "Prescription Opioid Use, Misuse, and Use Disorders in U.S. Adults: 2015 National Survey on Drug Use and Health." *Annals of Internal Medicine* 167 (5): 293–301.

Institute of Medicine (US) Committee on Advancing Pain Research, Care, and Education. 2011. *Relieving Pain in America: A Blueprint for Transforming*

Prevention, Care, Education, and Research. Washington, DC: National Academies Press.

John Paul II. 1987. Letter to pain specialists. July 27, 1987. International Association for the Study of Pain Records. Manuscript Collections no. 124. John C. Liebeskind History of Pain Collection, UCLA Library Special Collection.

Lasagna, L., and H. K. Beecher. 1954. "The Optimal Dose of Morphine." *JAMA* 156 (3): 230–34.

Melzack, R. 1990. "The Tragedy of Needless Pain." *Scientific American* 262 (2): 27–33.

Morpurgo, C. V., and D. N. Spinelli. 1976. "Plasticity of Pain Perception." *Brain Theory Newsletter* 2:14–15.

National Center for Injury Prevention and Control and Division of Unintentional Injury Prevention. 2011. "Policy Impact: Prescription Painkiller Overdoses." Atlanta: U.S. Department of Health and Human Services: CDC. Last accessed September 10, 2020. https://www.cdc .gov/drugoverdose/pdf/policyimpact -prescriptionpainkillerod-a.pdf.

National Institutes of Health. 2014. "Pathways to Prevention Workshop: The Role of Opioids in the Treatment of Chronic Pain." September 29–30, 2014. https:// prevention.nih.gov/sites/default/files /documents/programs/p2p/ODPPain PanelStatementFinal_10-02-14.pdf.

Page, G. G., S. Ben-Eliyahu, R. Yirmiya, and J. C. Liebeskind. 1993. "Morphine Attenuates Surgery-Induced Enhancement of Metastatic Colonization in Rats." *Pain* 54 (1): 21–28.

Panocka, I., P. Marek, and B. Sadowski. 1986. "Differentiation of Neurochemical Basis of Stress-Induced Analgesia in Mice by Selective Breeding." *Brain Research* 397 (1): 156–60.

Perry, M. J. 2017. "What the US Can Learn from Portugal's Drug Decriminalization." Foundation for Economic Education. July 14, 2017. https://fee.org/articles /what-the-us-can-learn-from-portugals -drug-decriminalization.

Petrosky, E., R. Harpaz, K. A. Fowler, M. K. Bohm, C. G. Helmick, K. Yuan, and C. J. Betz. 2018. "Chronic Pain Among

Suicide Decedents, 2003 to 2014: Findings from the National Violent Death Reporting System." *Annals of Internal Medicine* 169 (7): 448–55.

Ready, L. B., R. Oden, H. S. Chadwick, C. Benedetti, G. A. Rooke, R. Caplan, and L. M. Wild. 1988. "Development of an Anesthesiology-Based Postoperative Pain Management Service." *Anesthesiology* 68 (1): 100–106.

Rich, B. A. 2006. "The Ethical Dimensions of Pain and Suffering." In *Pain Management at the End of Life: Bridging the Gap Between Knowledge and Practice*, edited by K. J. Doka, 245–60. Living with Grief. Washington, DC: Hospice Foundation of America.

Richmond, C. 2005. "Dame Cicely Saunders." *British Medical Journal* 331 (7510): 238.

Rose, M. E. 2018. "Are Prescription Opioids Driving the Opioid Crisis? Assumptions vs Facts." *Pain Medicine* 19 (4): 793–807.

Scholl, L., P. Seth, M. Kariisa, N. Wilson, and G. Baldwin. 2019. "Drug and Opioid-Involved Overdose Deaths—United States, 2013–2017." *Morbidity and Mortality Weekly Report* 67 (5152): 1419–27.

Shipton, E. E., F. Bate, R. Garrick, C. Steketee, E. A. Shipton, and E. J. Visser. 2018. "Systematic Review of Pain Medicine Content, Teaching, and Assessment in Medical School Curricula Internationally." *Pain and Therapy* 7 (2): 139–61.

Singh, G. 1998. "Recent Considerations in Nonsteroidal Anti-Inflammatory Drug Gastropathy." *American Journal of Medicine* 105 (1B): 31S–38S.

Sullivan, D. R., B. Chan, J. A. Lapidus, L. Ganzini, L. Hansen, P. A. Carney, E. K. Fromme, M. Marino, S. E. Golden, K. C. Vranas, and C. G. Slatore. 2019. "Association of Early Palliative Care Use with Survival and Place of Death Among Patients with Advanced Lung Cancer Receiving Care in the Veterans Health Administration." *JAMA Oncology* 5 (12): 1702–9. https://doi.org/10.1001 /jamaoncol.2019.3105.

Temel, J. S., J. A. Greer, A. Muzikansky, E. R. Gallagher, S. Admane, V. A. Jackson, C. M. Dahlin, C. D. Blinderman, J.

Jacobsen, W. F., Pirl, J. A. Billings, and T. J. Lynch. 2010. "Early Palliative Care for Patients with Metastatic Non-Small-Cell Lung Cancer." *New England Journal of Medicine* 363:733–42.

U.S. Department of Health and Human Services Working Group on Patient-Centered Reduction or Discontinuation of Long-Term Opioid Analgesics. 2019. "HHS Guide for Clinicians on the Appropriate Dosage Reduction or Discontinuation of Long-Term Opioid Analgesics." October 2019. https://www.hhs.gov/opioids/sites/default/files/2019-10/Dosage_Reduction_Discontinuation.pdf.

Watt-Watson, J., M. McGillion, J. Hunter, M. Choiniere, A. J. Clark, A. Dewar, C. Johnston, M. Lynch, P. Morley-Forster,

D. Moulin, N. Thie, C. L. von Baeyer, and K. Webber. 2009. "A Survey of Prelicensure Pain Curricula in Health Science Faculties in Canadian Universities." *Pain Research and Management* 14 (6): 439–44.

Wee Jun Yan, I., B. Lim Tian Ying, and F. Brennan. 2018. "Public Policy: An Analgesia for Opioid Diversion." *Journal of Pain and Palliative Care Pharmacotherapy* 32 (2–3): 178–91.

Yeager, M. P., D. D. Glass, R. K. Neff, and T. Brinck-Johnsen. 1987. "Epidural Anesthesia and Analgesia in High-Risk Surgical Patients." *Anesthesiology* 66 (6): 729–36.

CHAPTER 12

Artificial Intelligence in Palliative Care

An Integral Look into the Future of Our End

Dominique J. Monlezun

In a cramped broom closet–become–conference room, I huddled beside a husband sobbing as I had to tell him his wife was dying. As the physician, my job was to apply the best of modern medicine to give her the best chance of surviving. But her liver infection had spread throughout her body so quickly that all the medicines, machines, and minutes pouring into her could not stop her from slipping away from us. "I am so sorry, but I have to ask, 'What would she want us to do?'" "I want her to live . . ." was the only answer he could give me.

Palliative care makes possible (and human) this difficult but needed conversation for those we lose quickly and those who have a little more time. It helps patients and their families achieve and maintain comfort amid the pain and other distress of the too often lonely journey toward death. In many ways, palliative care is one of the most human of all medicine's specialties, the most eminently aware of the limitations of our sciences, the most hopeful for the power of human companionship that supersedes our technological interventions with their material complexity, steps in the right direction to answer the immaterial questions of "how" and "why." And it was palliative care that steadied my voice and tears as I held that husband's hand and led him to his wife.

The intimate human spiritual connection of palliative care will always be essential, but what will be the impact of artificial intelligence (AI), which is driving the twenty-first century's technological explosion and so rapidly transforming both medicine and modern society? It is reasonable to assume that AI will make us smarter, faster, and better at curing disease, but will it yield similar improvements in comforting patients and creating hope? The potential advances of AI bring us to renewed metaphysical and philosophical questions. Is there an ethical or right way to use AI, particularly in palliative care, when we are facing the ultimate reminder of our human limitations, namely our deaths? Will AI make us even question who we are as human beings and what death means, such as in research attempting to extend the consciousness of people beyond death?

To understand how AI might impact palliative care, we need first to understand who we are (i.e., metaphysics), how AI works (i.e., its mathematics), and how it applies to palliative care (i.e., its medicine). AI comes from human intelligence, which is governed by human wisdom. Knowing "how" to give palliative drugs does not make one a physician; knowing the "why" based on biology (and its derivative pharmacology) is a step toward being one. So let us explore this "why" and "how" of AI palliative care through the three-rung ladder of its metaphysics, mathematics, and medicine. Hopefully, this shared climb will enable us to better understand how the technological intervention of AI might make palliative care even more human at one of our most human defining moments—our own deaths and the deaths of those whom we accompany.

METAPHYSICS AND AI PALLIATIVE CARE

Physicians cannot apply medicine to treat patients in the right clinical way without knowing biology (or the physics and chemistry that give rise to physical or material processes at the subatomic, atomic, cellular, and organ system level to give, sustain, or end life). Similarly, we cannot apply ethics to treat patients (even with AI's help) in the right way without some knowledge of philosophy, particularly metaphysics (or the study of being as being, and thus first principles or highest causes of all effects through which we alone can understand being). Why do we need to think about metaphysics? Because there are only two ways to resolve disagreements: politics or philosophy, might or right. Either you must be stronger than me, or we must agree on a common understanding to solve a disagreement. And this understanding is only reached through a common moral language enabled by and aiming at a common understanding of objective good. Metaphysics provides the ultimate justification or compelling defense for any argument as its foundation, making possible the subsequent application of formal logic, including a systematic accounting of valid arguments applied to true premises, then leading to valid conclusions.

Let us consider the practical reasons also for starting here. Power is fleeting, but truth is not. Some people subjectively believe (or have a self-defined belief created by referencing themselves instead of an external or objective standard) that, for instance, we should let AI decide who lives and dies based on social utility not just in palliative care but in population health. Such people, if they have enough power, can implement their belief. The only way sustainably to resist the above is if we are united by a common understanding of what the objective good is (i.e., every person has a right to her/his life and cannot be unjustly deprived of life because she/he has dignity as a unique individual). But many argue that the modern philosophy that dominates our laws and organizations says there is no such objective standard, for it follows the seventeenth-century European Enlightenment, which rejected any metaphysics, philosophy, or standard for understanding the world or right action higher than human rationality—you make your own truth. But what happens if each person's subjectively defined truth contradicts that of others? How might such conflict be resolved? Without a common moral language, the one who decides what we do is the one who has more power.

The modern German philosopher Friedrich Nietzsche (1844–1900) claimed that "God is dead. . . . And we have killed him."[1] Nietzsche believed that the inevitable consequence of the Enlightenment (making human rationality the ultimate philosophical standard) is this: there is nothing to stop us from realizing that there is no right or wrong, no good or evil, that we are own creators, our own gods, that there is only power or weakness. We should fight for power as the highest form or "good" of humanity. We know that the National Socialists (Nazis) saw themselves as the embodiment of Nietzsche's supermen, the strong who seized power from the weak by killing them, as this was their highest "good." Clearly, without good philosophy, politics has and will weaponize science and technology. Since AI has even more potential than military weapons—to create almost unimaginable evil—can we thus consider how *good* philosophy may make AI palliative care good?

Let us start with the Greek physician-philosopher Aristotle (384–322 BCE), who developed metaphysics to understand what it means for anything to be, including human beings. He observed that we exist with a particular essence as human beings, different from how a horse exists as a horse or a rock as a rock. And yet, unlike other things, humans are unique in that our human essence means we exist as a substantive union of matter and form, physically and nonphysically or spiritually. Do you say you love someone because you can quantify a sufficient oxytocin neuro-hormonal surge in your brain when that person walks in front of you, or is love deeper than the material but just as real? And Aristotle observed that something else, something higher is the cause or reason of why we exist. You were created by your parents, and your parents by their parents, and back and back through history. But eventually, as Aristotle argued, there must be some uncaused cause (for it is not logical to go on as such into infinity). In other words, you can see a rock rolling down a mountain, but it did not spontaneously move itself. Something else had to first move it (meaning there logically must be something that is the unmoved mover). Aristotle therefore concluded that metaphysics as the highest form of human knowledge arrives at its final destination of inquiry about the uncaused cause, or the divine; philosophy thus gives way to theology as humanity reaches to its furthest limits until it attempts to glimpse the limitless.

Later the Italian Catholic priest-philosopher Thomas Aquinas (1225–1274) integrated diverse cultures and thought-systems, from Aristotle to the Persian Muslim physician-philosopher Avicenna (980–1037) to the Spanish Jewish rabbi-philosopher Maimonides (1138–1204) in order ultimately to argue that this uncaused cause is God. Pulling from these diverse sources, Aquinas argued that God is also the supreme good, the highest truth, love itself, our ultimate cause and final end. Each human being created in God's image with intellect and free will naturally seeks to know and desire the good over evil (or its absence), as each person is drawn from within the depths of her/his being to God and thus into communion with this supreme good through whom the person finds completion and happiness. My patient was happiest being a wife and a mom; she loved being at the dinner table with her family because she loved them and found she was most herself by being with them. The more she knew them, the more she wanted to be with them, the more she became a wife and mother and thus herself, the happier or more fulfilled she became. According to Aquinas, each person therefore is made by love for love through love, and so each person naturally has dignity that no one should artificially limit. Each person has rights to things that are required for them to become happy by becoming good and reaching the supreme good. Each person has duties to contribute to the common good as the collective good of each person, protecting the dignity and so rights of each person. We exist as persons in communities of persons (our families, schools, businesses, states, etc.), and so we naturally know that we should do good and avoid evil as the only right or good way to interact with others who are also persons. Aquinas called this naturally known organic system of right relationships the "natural law," which is normative, telling us what we ought to do. Natural law in accordance with the supreme good makes justice possible.

A millennium later, the Polish Catholic pope-philosopher Karol Wojtyła, or John Paul II (1920–2005), integrated modern psychology with Thomistic-Aristotelian philosophy to observe that people everywhere, regardless of their age, sex, race, nation, socioeconomic status, religion (or lack thereof), abilities, and other characteristics, are all united in a global human family. We can and are meant to exist together in justice and peace—by understanding what it means to be a person (both intellectually and experientially): "Man cannot live without love. He remains a being that is incomprehensible for himself . . . if he does not experience it and make it his own."[2] And what is this love? "Love commits to freedom and imbues it with that to which the will is naturally attracted—goodness. . . . Man longs for love more than for freedom—freedom that is the means and love the end. . . . From the desire for the 'unlimited' good of another 'I' springs the whole creative drive of true love—the drive to endow beloved persons with the good, to make them happy. . . . To desire 'unlimited' good for another person is really to desire God for that person."[3]

Think of a time you told someone you loved that person. Did you not mean that you want that person's good, for her/him to be happy? In each person's particular historical moment and cultural context, within the person's understanding of the world and ultimate cause (God the Father, Son, and Holy Spirit; Allah; Yahweh; Brahma; a universal rationality that points to a unnamed power above us; etc.), do we as a pluralistic people of diverse beliefs not know in the depths of our hearts that there must be something bigger than us, an objective reality that makes our subjective experience of it possible? Do we not know that we are not our own creators nor our own gods? The presence of this pluralism does not prove that there is no universal objective good—it rather manifests that such a good must exist. As climbers beginning from different paths on a mountain all drawn in the same direction upward, so too diverse belief systems exist and converge on that unifying good at the metaphysical summit.

Modern philosophy unravels as it commits itself to a foundational logical fallacy by metaphysically claiming in a circular argument that there is no metaphysics, no higher reason than that which we create, no unifying good, no God. Wojtyła in his 1995 address to the United Nations (UN) General Assembly argued something different: "Every culture is an effort to ponder the mystery of the world and in particular of the human person: it is a way of giving expression to the transcendent dimension of human life. The heart of every culture is its approach to the greatest of all mysteries: the mystery of God."[4]

AI and palliative care necessarily express and are explained at least in part by the cultures within which they are embedded. Understanding them in their most basic function as collective and individual pursuits of the transcendental human mysteries, including the greatest mystery of the supreme good, may help us advance our understanding of them. And so let us turn back to Wojtyła's philosophy of Thomistic personalism and how it clarified or refined the modern philosophical structure of the UN's conception of human rights, dating back to its seminal formulation in the 1948 Universal Declaration of Human Rights (UDHR). This global vision and concrete commitment, established before the ash of the Nazi war crimes had time to settle, served as the common statement of the world's people about their belief in the dignity and thus rights of every person and states' duties to protect them. Under the leadership of the Lebanese Christian Thomistic philosopher-diplomat Charles Malik (1906–1987), who led as a UDHR Drafting Committee member and chair of the UN's Third Committee, which approved the *Declaration*, the UDHR was ratified for the same belief that opened it: "Whereas recognition of the inherent dignity and of the equal and inalienable rights of all members of the human family is the foundation of freedom, justice, and peace in the world . . . THE GENERAL ASSEMBLY proclaims THIS UNIVERSAL DECLARATION OF HUMAN RIGHTS as a common standard of achievement for all peoples and all nations."[5]

The UN, with its derivative international law and modern emphasis on rights, is not simply a social contract—it is personal communion, a personalist contract that commits itself to a metaphysical foundation articulated by Thomistic-Aristotelian natural law. The early UN president Carlos Romulo (1898–1985) argued that the UDHR "demonstrated most clearly . . . the tendency to work out a system of international law conforming as closely as possible to natural law," further arguing that "faithful adherence to Christian doctrine and the law of God has become a *sine qua non* of the survival of mankind."[6] Romulo, like Wojtyła, refined the UN's social contract of human rights through Christianity's Thomistic natural law, seeking to make natural law philosophically intelligible and defensible for pluralistic peoples, without making people become Christian.

But why bring all this up? Because the philosophical framework of UN rights is the world's only shared ethics (by virtue of every nation ratifying it and integrating it into their state governance and culture). And the natural law articulated by Wojtyła's Thomistic personalism may make it philosophically defensible and still intelligible to the world's various belief systems. AI is rapidly transforming our globalized world as a powerful tool for good or evil, especially if used to guide decisions about who is born, who lives, and who dies. Such a "personalist social contact" may provide a clear and compelling global bioethics of AI palliative care to enable a healing tool rather than a destructive weapon.

MATHEMATICS AND AI PALLIATIVE CARE

The above section focused on the theoretical or "why" behind AI palliative care. Now let us consider the material or applied dimension, the "how" of this topic. Among the 29 million+ biomedical citations catalogued in the PubMed online database by the United States National Institutes of Health's National Library of Medicine, only five, as of July 2019, focus on AI and palliative care and allow viewable abstracts. They all focus on improving quality metrics through faster identification of metrics, high-risk patients, or clinician competencies. Most of the citations feature AI in the form of machine learning (ML) algorithms.

In one study, a supervised ML algorithm was applied to one thousand randomly selected audio clips in clinician-patient serious illness discussions. ML had comparable performance but was 61 percent faster than manual human coding at identifying connectional silence, a core quality component.[7] Similarly, a study of breast cancer patients showed how natural language processing (NLP) was applied to the electronic medical record to quickly identify with 100 percent positive predictive value (PPV) those patients who have malignancy with particularly poor prognosis, thus prompting more targeted palliative interventions.[8] NLP was used in another study for rapid and accurate identification of medical students' geriatric competency exposures based on their clinical notes reflecting competencies in medical management, self-care capacity, hospital care for elders, and disorders of falls, balance, and gait.[9] A final traditional ML application was demonstrated in a single-center cohort study of a New York community palliative program in which a ML-based automated information system optimized clinician management of palliative care patients with personalized evidence-based recommendations specific for the particular patient.[10] There was one application of deep learning (a more advanced version of AI in which there is little if any human input so the algorithm can learn by itself from the data and so answer questions from it). It had nearly comparable performance to clinicians identifying patient preferences in the intensive care unit (ICU) but in drastically less time, allowing earlier discussions within forty-eight hours of ICU admission.[11]

MEDICINE AND AI PALLIATIVE CARE

Building on the above metaphysical and mathematical foundations, optimal AI palliative care may be defined as providing the most clinically effective, cost-effective, and equitable care for each person to enhance her/his chances of living as well as possible with serious illness and, when death does come, having a good death. The above studies highlight how AI may already be used to identify high-risk patients, the care they need, and how palliative care professionals might optimally care for them. Current AI palliative care may even assist with training the next generation of providers. But what else might AI palliative care offer in the near future?

Can AI palliative care, not just mathematically and medically but also metaphysically, promote palliative care in a holistic way that treats the patient as a person with the right treatment at the right time at the right cost? Recent research in population health more generally borrowing from demonstrated proof-of-concept applications in clinical medicine (with application for palliative care) suggests that near-term AI optimization of palliative care can plausibly focus on automated NLP approaches to accelerate timely diagnosis, with ML guiding real-time evidence-based recommendations to clinicians to treat a particular patient concurrently with identifying clusters of diseases of public health concern guiding population-level interventions.[12] Specific to palliative care, such a comprehensive approach could prevent expensive comorbidities through high-value (low cost, high clinical benefit) population health interventions[13] (such as cooking classes for families integrated with medical care),[14] particularly for lower-income patients who have difficulty affording medications and procedures and have lower health literacy recognizing symptoms of developing comorbidities. A ML system integrated into their electronic health record may notify clinicians about the likelihood and timing of catastrophic events and how to prevent such events through earlier interventions and also promote patient-centered end-of-life care plans for the time when prevention and treatment of serious illness ultimately fails, as it always must at some point for each of us as mortal beings.

CONCLUSION

I have tried to offer an integrated vision of the metaphysics, mathematics, and medicine of palliative care in the hope of better understanding the role AI is starting to play and will likely play even more in the future. AI has the potential to accelerate providers' capacity to personalize optimal palliative care for each patient as part of a continuum of optimal lifelong care, making it more equitable, effective, and human. Yet such a rosy scenario is not guaranteed, for I believe that AI without an appropriate metaphysical foundation has the potential for great harm, devaluing the very sanctity of life. To guard against such harm, I believe a Thomistic personalism as expressed via the UN's human rights social contract is essential to a morally good application of AI in palliative care. The declaration offers us a defensible, logical, and universal understanding of who we are as persons, what makes a good community, a good life, and ultimately a good death.

Death is inevitable, but the physical, emotional, social, and spiritual suffering of total pain is not. AI, appropriately applied to palliative care, can help ensure that each element of total pain is palliated to the best of our ability, augmented by the incredible power of machine learning focused on the good of each patient as a person. My patient and her husband, whom I described at the beginning of this essay, deserve this. We all do.

NOTES

1. Nietzsche 1991, section 125.
2. John Paul II 1979, section 10.
3. Wojtyła 1993, 135–38.

4. John Paul II 1995, section 9.
5. UNESCO 2005, preamble.
6. Romulo 1950, 123.

7. Durieux et al. 2018.
8. Udelsman et al. 2019.
9. Chen et al. 2014.
10. Tamang et al. 2005.

11. Chan et al. 2019.
12. Lavigne et al. 2019.
13. Monlezun et al. 2018.
14. Monlezun et al. 2015.

WORKS CITED

Chan, A., I. Chien, E. Moseley, S. Salman, S. Kaminer Bourland, D. Lamas, A. M. Walling, J. A. Tulsk, and C. Lindvall. 2019. "Deep Learning Algorithms to Identify Documentation of Serious Illness Conversations During Intensive Care Unit Admissions." *Palliative Medicine* 33 (2): 187–96. doi: 10.1177/0269216318810421.

Chen, Y., J. Wrenn, H. Xu, A. Spickard III, R. Habermann, J. Powers, and J. C. Denny. 2014. "Automated Assessment of Medical Students' Clinical Exposures According to AAMC Geriatric Competencies." *AMIA Annual Symposium Proceedings* 2014: 375–84.

Durieux, B. N., C. J. Gramling, V. Manukyan, M. J. Eppstein, D. M. Rizzo, L. M. Ross, A. G. Ryan, M. A. Niland, L. A. Clarfeld, S. C. Alexander, and R. Gramling. 2018. "Identifying *Connectional Silence* in Palliative Care Consultations: A Tandem Machine-Learning and Human Coding Method." *Journal of Palliative Medicine* 21 (12): 1755–60. doi: 10.1089/jpm.2018.0270.

John Paul II. 1979. "Redemptor Hominis." *The Holy See*, March 4, 1979. http://w2.vatican.va/content/john-paul-ii/en/encyclicals/documents/hf_jp-ii_enc_04031979_redemptor-hominis.html.

———. 1995. "Address of His Holiness John Paul II." Speech to the Fiftieth General Assembly of the United Nations Organization, New York, October 5, 1995. http://w2.vatican.va/content/john-paul-ii/en/speeches/1995/october/documents/hf_jp-ii_spe_05101995_address-to-uno.html.

———. *See also* Wojtyła, K.

Lavigne, M., R. Mussa, M. I. Creatore, S. J. Hoffman, and D. L. Buckeridge. 2019. "A Population Health Perspective on Artificial Intelligence." *Healthcare Management Forum* 32 (4): 173–77. doi: 10.1177/0840470419848428.

Monlezun, D. J. 2020. *The Global Bioethics of Artificial Intelligence and Human Rights*. Cambridge: Cambridge Scholars.

Monlezun, D. J., L. Dart, A. Vanbeber, P. Smith-Barbaro, V. Costilla, C. Samuel, C. A. Terregino, E. Ercikan Abali, B. Dollinger, N. Baumgartner, N. Kramer, A. Seelochan, S. Taher, M. Deutchman, M. Evans, R. B. Ellis, S. Oyola, G. Maker-Clark, T. Dreibelbis, I. Budnick, D. Tran, N. DeValle, R. Shepard, E. Chow, C. Petrin, A. Razavi, C. McGowan, A. Grant, M. Bird, C. Carry, G. McGowan, C. McCullough, C. M. Berman, K. Dotson, T. Niu, L. Sarris, and T. S. Harlan. 2018. "Machine Learning-Augmented Propensity Score-Adjusted Multilevel Mixed Effects Panel Analysis of Hands-On Cooking and Nutrition Education Versus Traditional Curriculum for Medical Students as Preventive Cardiology: Multisite Cohort Study of 3,248 Trainees over 5 Years." *BioMed Research International*. 2018: 5051289.

Monlezun, D. J., E. Kasprowicz, K. W. Tosh, J. Nix, P. Urday, D. Tice, L. Sarris, and T. S. Harlan. 2015. "Medical School-Based Teaching Kitchen Improves HbA1c, Blood Pressure, and Cholesterol for Patients with Type 2 Diabetes: Results from a Novel Randomized Controlled Trial." *Diabetes Research and Clinical Practice* 109 (2): 420–26.

Nietzsche, F. 1991. *The Gay Science*. 1882. Translated by W. Kaufmann. New York: Random House.

Rawls, J. 1999. *A Theory of Justice*. Rev. ed. Cambridge, MA: Harvard University Press.

Romulo, C. P. 1950. "Natural Law and International Law." In *Natural Law*

Institute Proceedings, vol. 3, edited by E. F. Barrett, 119–28. Notre Dame: College of Law, University of Notre Dame.

Tamang, S., D. Kopec, G. Shagas, and K. Levy. 2005. "Improving End of Life Care: An Information Systems Approach to Reducing Medical Errors." *Studies in Health Technology and Informatics* 114:93–104.

Udelsman, B., I. Chien, K. Ouchi, K. Brizzi, J. A. Tulsky, and C. Lindvall. 2019. "Needle in a Haystack: Natural Language Processing to Identify Serious Illness." *Journal of Palliative Medicine* 22 (2): 179–82. doi: 10.1089/jpm.2018.0294.

United Nations Educational, Scientific, and Cultural Organization. 2005. "Universal Declaration on Bioethics and Human Rights: Records of the General Conference." Paris, October 3–21, 2005. http://unesdoc.unesco.org.

Wojtyła, K. 1993. *Love and Responsibility*. Rev. ed. San Francisco: Ignatius.

———. *See also* John Paul II.

Palliative Care

The Caregiver

CHAPTER 13

A Spiritual Environment of Caring

Courtenay R. Bruce, Stacy L. Auld, and Charles R. Millikan

I was a newly minted chaplain. I just got hired on. And, sure, I worked in hospital wards before, and I thought I understood the needs of patients. Maybe I was just naïve. Or young and inexperienced. I don't know. Anyway, [I walked into] the room of a patient who was dying. She was alone. No family there. She had a [do-not-resuscitate order] in place, and the team was contemplating [withdrawing] the ventilator for a compassionate extubation to allow her to die from her underlying, very metastatic cancer to the bone, lung, liver . . . everything. I thought I would just do a prayer, right? I wanted to get in and get out. But I saw this look on her face. I wish I could describe it. It was a look of sadness and death, for sure. But there was something else there. A look of . . . uncertainty. Of fright. So I tried to figure out how to communicate with her, because I desperately wanted to figure out why she looked scared. Anyway, with the help of a communication board, pen and paper, and a super-patient nurse who helped me, I learned that the patient had done something really bad, I mean really bad, in her past. And she was scared to die, because she was afraid she wouldn't "see her family and God." I was able to talk with her about grace, forgiveness, love, guilt, heaven, reconciliation, her faith . . . over the next week in several brief meetings. One morning, I learned she passed peacefully. I hadn't finished my work with her, but she felt complete, I think, because she was holding her Bible when she died, and I heard she had a small tear in her eye. Not sadness. Relief. (From a senior chaplain in the Houston, Texas, area [edited to preserve anonymity])

This is just one story among thousands that illustrate how profoundly spiritual practices and beliefs impact how patients make decisions about treatment options and end-of-life care.[1] Other stories, coupled with compelling data, demonstrate how spiritual beliefs are positively associated with better health and psychological well-being. Patients themselves often reference their faith as a means of coping and healing.[2] Faith can provide a sense of meaning and purpose, as patients face serious illness.

United Methodists have long recognized the link between spirituality and medicine, as demonstrated widely in their church teachings.[3] For instance, United Methodists have consistently believed that the provision of health care for all patients without regard to status or ability to pay is integral to the Christian faith. John Wesley offered medical services at no cost to those individuals who were unable to pay, and the United Methodist Church urges its members to become actively involved at all levels in the development of health care systems for its community.[4] In this essay, we will offer insight into the ways in which Houston Methodist Hospital attempts to address the indissoluble link that exists between spirituality and patient care.

THE CONTEXT: HOUSTON METHODIST HOSPITAL

Houston Methodist Hospital (HMH) is a Christian organization established by the Texas Annual Conference of the United Methodist Church.[5] With over one thousand beds, HMH is the largest hospital in the system. From the start, HMH has had a strong faith-based ministry. Purchased by the Texas Annual Conference of the United Methodist Church from Dr. Oscar Norsworthy following World War I, HMH regarded itself as an extension of the church, yet with openness to all persons—of faith or no faith at all. Early on, the *I CARE Values* were initiated. This acronym, comprised by the words Integrity, Compassion, Accountability, Respect, and Excellence, marked an effort to motivate the entire hospital's work force toward a culture that represents these values.

In 2010, we, along with several other people, undertook several formative steps that we contend helped cement the permanent relationship between Methodism and patient care. One of the first initiatives consisted of writing a crisp mission statement and a values statement that explicitly named spirituality as a central tenet of hospital practices. HMH's mission statement now reflects that HMH provides high-quality, cost-effective health care to patients in a *spiritual* environment of caring in association with internationally recognized teaching and research. HMH's value statements explicate what it means to have a spiritual environment of caring informed by core Methodist values. For example, "we embrace the whole person and respond to emotional, ethical, and spiritual concerns as well as physical needs."[6]

THE INTEGRATION OF SPIRITUALITY AT HOUSTON METHODIST HOSPITAL

Integrating spirituality within hospital walls required more than a mission and values statement. Therefore, we used a phased approach to become more integrated incrementally throughout the system. We chose the word "embed" to describe the phased-approach intervention for increased integration because it highlights the importance of sustained and close contacts with a particular practice setting and its personnel, patients, and families.[7] Embedding spirituality would allow spiritual leaders to become part of clinical units or with specialty teams. With routine presence and interactions, they would have, it was hoped, enhanced opportunities to gain information, form relationships, and enhance their contributions.

Phase One: The Integration of Spirituality

During the first phase of the embedding process, we participated in hospital committee meetings, such as health care executive leadership committee meetings, institutional review board meetings, and medical executive committee meetings. We believed that it was not enough to be present during the meetings; we instead opted for a more active approach by becoming integral to decision-making processes.

To become "accepted" at leadership meetings, we knew it would be critical to gain the respect of physicians and administrators alike. Thus, we would meet with physicians in order to learn more about their perspectives on chaplaincy and spirituality in medicine. We would ask what chaplaincy could do to help them so that we would be "invited in," rather than having to dogmatically "assert" our presence and participation. Physicians often reported that they thought it would be helpful if chaplaincy could help identify patients' spiritual needs proactively, so we offered to attend clinical meetings and rounds to learn more about patients' spiritual needs. We showed administration that we could independently seek funding by securing additional funding for chaplaincy needs through philanthropy. By demonstrating that we would look for alternative ways of funding, we were able to show a sincere commitment to our notion of faith and healing and its role in good patient care, which conveyed a level of seriousness and authenticity that administration needed to fully accept our inclusion in leadership meetings.

After we became a "known" figure, our involvement in leadership meetings became more standardized. Specifically, we began committee meetings with a five-minute reflection, encouraging hospital leadership to pause and reflect on the greater good, health and well-being, and positive thinking. During committee deliberations, we would remind leadership to maintain integrity in their decision-making processes by, for example, ensuring that like cases were treated similarly and that, where a different outcome was reached on a case, it was because of a legitimate ethical consideration that warranted a different mode of analysis as opposed to treating financial considerations as continuously paramount. By participating in committee discussions, we helped to ensure systematic, transparent, and equitable decision-making in a way that would fully respect the United Methodist Church's teachings. We also encouraged a chaplaincy consult, where appropriate, and reminded committee members to think about spiritual needs and other nonmedical factors that influence patient care.

Phase Two: The Growth of Spiritual Care Personnel

During the second part of the phased-in approach for increased integration, we hired more chaplains to become integrated in different aspects of the patient experience. In order to receive financial support for additional chaplaincy hiring, we knew it would be important to "speak the same language" as health care administrators and managers. That is, administrators generally think in terms of outcomes-centered evaluative strategies, like cost reductions or shortened length of stay. Spirituality is not especially amenable to quantification in the same way as cost reductions or lengths of stay. We met this challenge by quantifying our services in a way that was amenable to hospital administrators.

To quantify "spiritual care needs," we monitored patient and employee satisfaction scores. To monitor chaplains' effectiveness, we added a spiritual care question to patient and employee satisfaction surveys. Results from those surveys indicated that it would be necessary to offer chaplaincy services full-time, seven days a week, twenty-four hours a day. To provide these services, several contract chaplains were hired to give assistance to the full-time chaplains on staff. The number of chaplains grew from a handful to eighty-five. Each hospital would have its own director for spiritual care and a unit of chaplaincy care volunteers to assist in patient visits. These volunteers were vetted through the human resources department and its department of volunteers.

In addition to traditional chaplaincy positions related to service lines, HMH's Department of Spiritual Care employs a chaplain to the workplace, which serves employees who do not have any patient contact; a chaplain to physicians; and a chaplain to the palliative and supportive care service. Also, a system director has been added to assist the vice president to ensure that the spiritual care offices throughout the network hospital are properly coordinated and function as a system.

Additionally, we started collecting and routinely reporting other metrics, including spiritual care visits. Currently, about two hundred and fifty thousand visits are made annually, with 30 percent being made by the chaplaincy care volunteers. In 2018, we realized that only reporting the number of visits resulted in an incomprehensive picture of our ministry, so in addition to these metrics, we now report the number of staff support interactions, values integration efforts, and education events hosted for the wider community.

With that being said, the field of chaplaincy continues to struggle with knowing what is meaningful to report, especially what might be meaningful to hospital executives. Currently, we set targets for how many patients we visit prior to surgery and how many patients we visit in the emergency department because internally we have deemed those areas high-impact areas. In January of 2020, we added a reporting metric in our electronic medical record documentation that captures the time spent with a patient. We know that time spent does not always translate to higher-quality interactions, but we are hopeful that it will give us some insight to establish additional targets.

Phase Three: Spirituality, Death, and Dying

The United Methodist Church expects its hospitals to provide ministry to those who are ill and dying.[8] This sort of ministry requires hospital employees to demonstrate practically and overtly the love and compassion of God through their loving presence, their listening, their kindness, and their respect for patients and their families.[9] Respecting patients and their families requires chaplains to be available to attend to the grief of patients and their families before death, emotional angst and suffering in the wake of death or dying, and the spiritual needs of patients and their families (e.g., a lack of closure at the end of life).

Consequently, the third and final phase of the embedding process involved focused efforts on a compassionate dying process for all patients. We referred to the United Methodist *Book of Discipline* as a point of reference for how to die well: the dying process, we argued, should be as compassionate as possible, requiring maximum comfort-care measures to alleviate all forms of suffering, which the *Book of Discipline* supports.[10] Moreover, life-supporting measures could be withdrawn or withheld where they only increased suffering or unnecessarily prolonged the dying process (and where the burdens of disease became all-consuming and refractory to treatment).[11] Dying should involve maximum care and support, with the patient surrounded by people who can love and care for them.

ENHANCING THE PROCESS OF DEATH: CONCRETE STRATEGIES

This phased approach to the integration of spirituality could have been left underdeveloped. We chose instead to offer specific strategies, particularly with respect to the process of dying. Therefore, within the last decade, we developed several initiatives to enhance the dying process.

1. No One Dies Alone (NODA)

No One Dies Alone (NODA) was one of our first initiatives related to death and dying.[12] Implemented at HMH in April 2007, NODA was a specific initiative created to ensure that the dying process would involve maximum care and support. Modeled after the originating NODA program founded by Sandra Clarke, RN, at Sacred Heart Medical Center, in Eugene, Oregon, volunteers (Compassionate Companions) are trained to sit with patients who are dying and who do not have family or available friends. One aspect of the program is a resource bag that contains sacred texts, poetry books, a hymnbook, and a portable music device with soft music. Early on in the program, HMH averaged four patients a year who died with a compassionate companion present. The relatively few referrals for this program likely reflect the demographics of HMH patients; most patients have at least one person who accompanies them in their final days. However, as long as one person would die alone, we remain committed to NODA.

This expression of compassion toward dying patients can help not only patients, families, and friends but also support staff who feel powerless because they know their patient is dying without a companion while staff attend to other patients. One chaplain relayed that she will never forget seeing a compassionate companion holding a patient's hand and singing softly. She stopped at the window outside the patient's door, right as the patient took her last breath. The chaplain watched as the companion remained beside the patient as the patient died. Afterward, that chaplain asked the companion about her experience during the patient's passing. The companion replied, "It was so sacred; I was not able to be there with my mom when she died, but I am glad I was able to be there with this woman. She was not alone, and, in some ways, that's healing for me too."

2. Death and Dying Guidelines to Ensure Cultural Sensitivity

A second initiative involved ensuring that the dying process would be culturally sensitive and equitable. In 2015, we created guidelines to care for Jewish, Muslim, and Hindu patients. In collaboration with our faith leaders in the Houston community, we, along with many other chaplains from neighboring hospitals in the Texas Medical Center, created a one-page resource for each respective faith tradition that included specific religious protocols for how to handle a deceased person's body, suggested prayers or readings to use at the time of death, and phone numbers for religious leaders in the community.

One chaplain reported that, through the development of these guidelines, he felt more confident in leading the care team through the dying process of a Muslim patient who, in Houston for business, became ill and died suddenly during hospitalization. A couple of colleagues were with the patient, but he did not have family members present. The chaplain reported that, because of his familiarity with the guidelines, he was able to assure the off-site family on the phone that the body was being cared for respectfully. For example, it was positioned toward Mecca while the care team waited for a faith leader from the Islamic Society of Greater Houston to arrive.

3. A Professional Chaplain for Palliative and Supportive Care Services

A third initiative developed to enhance the dying process was to foster a collaborative relationship with the palliative and supportive care service (PSCS). For many years, the PSCS made referrals for the chaplain to be a part of end-of-life decision-making conversations, but HMH began to encourage even greater collaboration between the PSCS and chaplaincy.

According the *Clinical Practice Guidelines for Quality Palliative Care* (4th ed.), published by the National Coalition for Hospice and Palliative Care, eight domains should be addressed in a high-quality PSCS.[13] Domain 5 speaks specifically to the spiritual, religious, and existential aspects of care, which professional chaplains are trained to address. Domain 7 speaks to the care of the patient nearing the end of life; this is typically within the scope of professional chaplains' responsibilities. These guidelines, coupled with other real-life evidence,[14] indicate that the input of a professional chaplain is necessary for adequate PSCS.[15]

Therefore, in January 2019, HMH dedicated a full-time chaplain exclusively to the PSCS. This palliative care chaplain connects and establishes a relationship with the patient and family. The palliative care chaplain then takes a targeted approach to facilitating a life review in an effort to elicit information regarding family dynamics, places of distress, and, ultimately, hopes and future plans for how to live out the reminder of their lives, no matter the duration.[16] By asking pointed questions like "Do you have a pain in your soul?" the palliative care chaplain can discern whether the patient has come to a place of acceptance about his or her illness and can embrace a good death. The palliative care chaplain nurtures and empowers the patient, while also encouraging the patient to experience liberation and reconciliation when needed.

4. An Ethics Consultation Service

A fourth initiative to enhance the dying process was to strengthen the ethics consultation service. Dying well should involve professional guidance to resolve ethical conflicts or ethical uncertainty.[17] To that end, we worked with the Center for Medical Ethics and Health Policy at the Baylor College of Medicine to make ethics consultants available to work inside HMH in some of its most sensitive areas. Their primary responsibility is to address value-laden conflict between family members or between family members and clinicians about end-of-life care, including life-sustaining treatment decisions.[18] Within months of their involvement within HMH walls, consults for assistance with end-of-life matters rose from 65 consults annually to over 150. For the last seven years, the ethics consultation service has maintained a consistent volume of 500 ethics consultations annually.

THE UNIQUE CHALLENGES OF A PALLIATIVE CARE CHAPLAIN

The third initiative, to install a chaplain at HMH specifically devoted to palliative care, has provided a unique set of challenges. For example, many patients with whom the HMH palliative care chaplain interacts are in the dying process. As such, it can be challenging for patients to communicate, either by virtue of mechanical assistance, such as ventilators, or because of the absence of physical strength that often accompanies the progression of disease. "I often find that I want to move the conversation along, if only to help ease the patient," she admits, "but, if I move the conversation along too quickly, I could make unwarranted inferences or assumptions, accidentally putting words into the patient's mouth. So I literally have to go piece-by-piece, asking for assurances from the patient that I correctly interpreted what they are thinking or feeling."

Another unique challenge palliative care chaplains experience is the variety of misunderstandings associated with the term "palliative" care. Often this is taken to mean that death is necessarily near. In reality, palliative care chaplains may be called upon to aid a patient's spiritual angst, even in situations where death may not be imminent. A palliative care chaplain in a neighboring hospital has spoken to this challenge: "If I introduce myself to the patient or family as a palliative care chaplain, I've already shut the door." He explains that many people think of hospice when they hear the words "palliative care." While palliative care chaplains do meet with patients who are dying, many other patients are not dying and may instead be experiencing existential suffering manifested in physical pain. To introduce himself in these situations, this chaplain begins by saying he would like for the patient to explore stress-ors in his or her life and how those stressors might have an impact upon his or her health. By approaching the topic broadly and generically (such as using innocuous terms like "stressors" rather than value-laden terms such as "suffer-ing" or "existential"), he finds patients are much more willing to talk; he, in turn, is able to elicit a helpful, structured narrative that allows him to target interventions and address patient needs.

A final barrier that palliative care chaplains experience—perhaps at a rate unlike other chaplains—is that they must build rapport quickly and appro-priately with the patient and family in order to make a meaningful impact. While all chaplains are charged with eliciting patients' spiritual preferences and needs, they often have the opportunity to build a therapeutic relation-ship over the course of several visits. A palliative care chaplain may not have the luxury of time. And while other chaplains may be called upon to address many different needs, ranging from prayer for a good recovery after surgery to existential crises, palliative care chaplains are most invariably called upon to assist where there is profound grief, suffering, or loss at issue. There are no light cases, sporadically intertwined throughout their day, to create a sense of respite. All of their patients require careful attention to the emotional cues and dynamics of others, and chaplains must discern accurately and efficiently.

Despite these challenges, palliative care chaplains (and other professionals who work with patients and families at the end of life) often report that their ability to help patients, families, and clinical teams to develop a way forward is one of the greatest gifts health care professionals have to offer. This is our experience as well. One of us was facilitating end-of-life conversations in an intensive care unit conference room with a patient's family and several health care professionals when the "code blue" sirens started. The patient who was the subject of our family meeting had experienced a cardiac arrest and died. When we returned to the ICU conference room to talk with the patient's wife about the passing of her husband, the patient's wife grabbed one of us and uttered a most agonizing, guttural cry. She then lamented, "How am I sup-posed to go home? How am I supposed to leave here without the man I was married to for sixty-two years? How do I do this alone? I don't know how to drive a car. I don't know how to replace a lightbulb." We knew there were no words at that moment to ease the pain. So we just sat there. For hours. Family members came and left, and she was finally strong enough to go home with the support of family and friends. Several months later, we ran into the patient's wife again. She instantly remembered who were and thanked us for being with her during the worst moments of her life. To us, it was a joy. To be with patients, families, and health care professionals during the most stressful and agonizing time of their lives is one of the greatest gifts we can offer as health care professionals at Houston Methodist Hospital.

NOTES

1. Puchalski 2004, 2001; Carpenter et al. 2008; Gryschek et al. 2019.

2. Puchalski 2004, 2001; Carpenter 2008; Gryschek et al. 2019.

3. United Methodist Church 2012.

4. Ibid.

5. "What We Believe" n.d.

6. Ibid.

7. Merriam-Webster online, s.v. "embed."

8. United Methodist Church 2012.

9. "What We Believe" n.d.

10. United Methodist Church 2016.

11. Ibid.

12. Kessler 2008.

13. Ibid.

14. Lawton 2000.

15. "Big Questions About Death" n.d.

16. Ibid.

17. Aulisio, Arnold, and Youngner 2000; Bliss et al. 2016; Dubler and Blustein 2007.

18. Aulisio, Arnold, and Youngner 1999.

WORKS CITED

Aulisio, M. P., R. M. Arnold, and S. J. Youngner. 1999. "An Ongoing Conversation: The Task Force Report and Bioethics Consultation." *Journal of Clinical Ethics* 10 (1): 3–4.

———. 2000. "Health Care Ethics Consultation: Nature, Goals, and Competencies: A Position Paper from the Society for Health and Human Values—Society for Bioethics Consultation Task Force on Standards for Bioethics Consultation." *Annals of Internal Medicine* 133 (1): 59–69.

"Big Questions About Death." n.d. *The Art of Dying Well.* St. Mary's University. Accessed September 11, 2019. https://www.artofdyingwell.org/what-is-dying-well/spiritual-questions/big-questions-death.

Bliss, S. E., J. Oppenlander, J. M. Dahlke, G. J. Meyer, E. M. Williford, and R. C. Macauley. 2016. "Measuring Quality in Ethics Consultation." *Journal of Clinical Ethics* 27 (2): 163–75.

Carpenter, K., L. Girvin, W. Kitner, and L. A. Ruth-Sahd. 2008. "Spirituality: A Dimension of Holistic Critical Care Nursing." *Dimensions of Critical Care Nursing* 27 (1): 16–20.

Dubler, N. N., and J. Blustein. 2007. "Credentialing Ethics Consultants: An Invitation to Collaboration." *American Journal of Bioethics* 7 (2): 35–37.

Ferrell, B. R., M. L. Twaddle, A. Melnick, and D. E. Meier. 2018. "National Consensus Project: Clinical Practice Guidelines for Quality Palliative Care." *Journal of Palliative Medicine* 21 (12): 1684–89.

Gryschek, G., D. A. Machado, L. J. Otuyama, C. Goodwin, and M. C. P. Lima. 2019. "Spiritual Coping and Psychological Symptoms as the End Approaches: A Closer Look on Ambulatory Palliative Care Patients." *Psychology, Health and Medicine* 25 (4): 426–33.

Kessler, L. 2008. "The Kindness of Strangers." Oprah.com, May 2008. Accessed August 22, 2019. https://www.oprah.com/omagazine/kindness-of-strangers-how-one-nurse-made-sure-no-one-dies-alone/all.

Lawton, J. 2000. *The Dying Process: Patients' Experiences with Palliative Care.* New York: Routledge.

Puchalski, C. M. 2001. "The Role of Spirituality in Health Care." *Baylor University Medical Center Proceedings* 14 (4): 352–57.

———. 2004. "Spirituality in Health: The Role of Spirituality in Critical Care." *Critical Care Clinics* 20 (3): 487–504.

United Methodist Church. 2012. *Book of Resolutions: Health and Wholeness.* Nashville: United Methodist Publishing House.

———. 2016. *Book of Discipline.* Nashville: United Methodist Publishing House.

"What We Believe." n.d. Houston Methodist Hospital. Accessed September 21, 2020. https://www.houstonmethodist.org/about-us/what-we-believe.

CHAPTER 14

Preparing Spiritual Caregivers

*Personal Reflections, Practical
Advice, and Helpful Programs*

W. Andrew Achenbaum

I am a historian and researcher on aging by profession and have spent most of my career at the interface between the humanities and medical science. I have had more opportunities to teach, observe, and learn from medical professionals than most persons outside of the healing professions will ever have. I have been challenged by and continue to learn from one particular case more than any other, and in this essay I will reflect on personal lessons learned related to the role of spirituality in caregiving.

The specific case in question involved a patient who spent more than ten weeks hospitalized with near constant pain, vomiting, dehydration, and infection complicating the treatment of cancer. She feared for her life but perhaps even more so for her autonomy, her sense of control, as she was moved from one unit to another, one test to another, one intervention to another, all in a desperate effort to save her life. "Will she die?" I asked the oncologist, who replied, "Time will tell." The response was honest, straightforward, yet uninformative and particularly frightening to me, for the patient and I had just married two months before hospitalization.

Decades of teaching courses on history and aging, discussing the book of Job and *The Death of Ivan Ilych*, and writing peer-reviewed books and essays had not prepared me to deal with the threat to my spouse's mortality, nor our mutual mental anguish and spiritual pain. I felt lost. Even though I received medical updates about my wife's condition, guidance for me as a caretaker was missing. For that I turned to Texas Medical Center (TMC) colleagues whom most persons would not have easy access to, including a spiritual care director and a psychotherapist. Otherwise, like most laypersons thrust into the role of caregiving, I turned to the internet. Roughly 87 percent of informal caregivers must figure out what to do by searching websites or reading newspapers; 61 percent claim that friends' suggestions and feedback from medical professionals prove insufficient.[1]

As a caretaker, I remain a work in progress—humbled by day-to-day challenges while harboring doubts about being good enough. Like many other caregivers whom I have met, I still feel quite unprepared for the task, yet I write this essay to provide health care professionals a brief overview of challenges faced by informal caretakers as well as to offer such caretakers some of my personal reflections in hopes of guiding them through caretaking, much as one might guide a traveler through "a foreign country with an unknown language."[2]

THE SCOPE OF CAREGIVING IN THE UNITED STATES

Most caregiving in America is performed by untrained individuals like me. Between 40 and 65 million Americans help elders; 15.7 million aid someone with Alzheimer's disease or a related dementia. While 70–75 percent of US caregivers are women, men also perform vital caregiving tasks.[3] Caregivers often face dual roles in a family, with a quarter of the middle-aged caregivers also raising children and juggling jobs, leading at least some to drop out of the workforce.[4] Almost 10 percent of caregivers are over age seventy-five, caring for aged peers, but young people also serve as caregivers, with 6 percent of Gen Z and 23 percent of millennials assisting someone with two or more debilitating conditions.[5]

Most caregivers devote at least twenty-five hours per week to the task, and some work round the clock; nearly 30 percent have been doing unpaid work for more than five years.[6] Caregiver tasks are diverse, including but not limited to either assisting with or entirely performing daily tasks of living such as meal preparation (sometimes of special diets), feeding, bathing, toileting, clothing, and medication management.[7] Perhaps most commonly, caregivers listen, talk, and provide companionship.

Informal caregiving takes a huge financial toll on 68 percent of family caregivers supporting loved ones. To cover living expenses, 63 percent withdrew money from savings; 21 percent borrowed money to provide care.[8] The economic value of informal caregiving was estimated in 2013 in excess of $470 billion—a total roughly equivalent to Walmart's sales that year, and a sum far exceeding paid home care or the total spending on Medicaid.[9]

Caregiving is also physically and emotionally taxing. Some gerontologists report that family caregivers have poorer physical health than comparable noncaregiving persons, but other data contradict the belief that caregiving increases mortality risks.[10]

My personal journey as a caregiver has mirrored much of what is described in the literature. Although I have avoided personal financial hardship, I have experienced physical strain and mental burnout. I have endured episodes of depression, grief, rage, anxiety, and stress—symptoms a large majority of family caregivers report.[11] I also have reconfigured social relationships—as do 62 percent of caregivers, who admit making difficult choices between spending time with friends and providing care.[12] In facing that challenge, I have come to realize that I cannot be all things to all people. Unless I set boundaries intentionally, I invariably become drained and disconnected.

THE IMPORTANCE OF SPIRITUAL CAREGIVING

"Where is the soul of evidence-based medicine?" psychotherapist Thomas Moore asks.[13] The question is paramount to me as one who works professionally in the world of evidence-based medicine but who is also religious and spiritual by nature. For me, prayer opens avenues to search for meaning and authenticity in the whirlwind of confusion. Faith centers me between polarities of duty and loneliness, where joy and regret meet. Spiritual caregiving is a grace-filled act. It engenders warmth and compassion. Exercising this gift in love, I believe, complements the healing powers of a surgeon's knife or the pharmacist's drugs. Grace-filled acts of profound caregiving may not effect a cure, but in my experience, when accompanied by evidence-based medicine, they enhance quality of life for patient and caregiver alike. In the remainder of this essay, I will focus on concepts that have guided my own spiritual journey as a caregiver and that might succor others who serve in this way.

The notion that spirituality might have a major impact on health is not new. Indeed, TMC created the Institute for Religion and Health in 1955 to sensitize physicians, nurses, and chaplains to and train them on the spiritual needs of patients.[14] Behavioral and social scientists have documented largely positive ties between spirituality, religion, and aging.[15] Researchers have designed and tested qualitative and quantitative tools to help integrate spirituality and religion into curricula for health care professionals and clinical practices.[16] Major US hospitals address patients' spiritual concerns in delivering integrative health care. The American Public Health Association, the National Association of Social Workers, the American Nurses Association, and the Association of American Medical Colleges (among others) uphold the right of competent terminally ill patients to receive spiritual support.[17] Patients' memoirs and blogs celebrate the benefits of this holistic approach to assuaging spiritual anguish.

Interdisciplinary teams in hospitals now make considerable efforts to incorporate spirituality into medical care, yet only half of hospitalized patients state that they were invited to talk about their deepest spiritual concerns, to make prayer part of daily medical rounds, or to ask members of their faith community to visit.[18] "The medical model in general—the way we interpret pain and suffering through the language of pathology, prognosis, epidemiology, treatment, and cure—absolutely dominates modern biomedicine and leads to this heavily instrumentalized understanding of human suffering," asserts Warren Kinghorn, MD, ThD.[19] It is not surprising, then, that breaches can occur within proactive spiritual protocols.

In this essay, however, I am more disturbed by another communication gap: too often, health care professionals preclude opportunities for caregivers like me to prepare ourselves spiritually to relieve patients' distress and pain. The research literature is scant but revealing.[20] My TMC colleagues have assessed spirituality, religiosity, and spiritual pain among informal caregivers.[21] Researchers elsewhere have formulated psychometric analyses to inventory volunteer caretakers' unmet spiritual needs.[22] Nonetheless, caregivers' confusion, fears, and difficulties sustaining relationships with spouses, children, or friends are too often overlooked.

Ignoring caregivers' spiritual needs and bonds to patients entails a huge price. Suffering does not cease when medical interventions in hospitals end. Many caregivers—even those like me who find extending patience and love to be rewarding and satisfying—stumble on the job and wish that they could give up. My own psychological signs of spiritual burnout include irritability and overreacting to mistakes and criticism. I am torn when friends recuperating from surgeries or former students coping with addictions ask me to be there for them. If I say yes, I often resent the imposition. If I say no, I castigate myself for choosing self-care and personal compassion over responding generously to their needs.

There is no simple, one-size-fits-all solution to such feelings, but there are a tremendous number of resources one might consult. In my own journey into caregiving, I frankly was amazed by the abundance and reported efficacy of available resources. So I proceed with sharing, hoping to reach caregivers who want advice when they encounter barriers in offering care.

HELPFUL RESOURCES FOR SPIRITUAL CAREGIVERS

Spiritual caregiving has prosaic aspects. There is wisdom in practicing self-care; in fact, the caregiver who does not engage in self-care may soon find themselves unable to provide care to others. In practical terms, this means maintaining good personal health habits such as a healthy diet, drinking plenty of water, exercising, and obtaining adequate sleep. Carving out a little personal time, having a hobby, and contacting friends can mitigate dis-ease about caregiving for a loved one with serious disease. Using carved out personal time for mind-body practices like Transcendental Meditation or yoga can help reduce negativity and enable caregivers to recover energy, calmness, purposefulness, and satisfaction.[23]

During my stint as a caregiver, I discovered that daily adherence to self-healing activities promoted my spiritual well-being. Meditating, mindfully breathing, and embracing an existential component to caregiving were an essential first step.

Choosing a transformative avenue through conscious awareness allows the possibility of grace, even if such transcendent moments do not always arise. Engaging the process of conscious meditation means accepting that I am not ultimately in charge. Instead, I must imagine a mysteriously ontological change of persona: I imagine serendipitously, perhaps symbolically, being connected to a Creator who beckons an escape from the morass—*if* I am willing to surrender ego to selfhood.

I do not presume to understand the science or Tao behind this metanoia. And yet, I have learned through practice that it works (sometimes) to stimulate humility, allowing gratitude and forgiveness to displace my perfectionism. While meditative practices, prayer, or a spiritual relationship with one's God may help some caregivers, such practices will not likely help all.

Moving beyond prayer, meditation, and mindfulness practices, I have also learned to rely on volunteer support teams to bolster my aptitude and attitude about informal caregiving. If I need a break, I ask friends to step in. Should more assistance be required, I can turn to adult day care programs in my neighborhood. (If no meeting places are available near you, the US Administration on Aging offers an Eldercare Locator as a public service.)[24] Most metropolitan areas have respite-care facilities, where professionally trained attendants can care for the patient and allow the family caregiver to rebalance and revitalize their life. Such programs can provide safe sites for caregivers to talk to peers about their circumstances. Exchanging stories and attaining spiritual support hearkens back to premises set forth in Alcoholic Anonymous, yet unlike AA, these programs do not require belief in a higher power as a precondition for participation.[25]

Some caregivers comb the yellow pages and search on Google for spiritual therapists who offer psychosocial interventions and meaning-centered psychotherapies.[26] (This mode of support, I note, is utilized by 30 percent of the therapists, who themselves become vicariously traumatized while addressing the spiritual needs of caregivers that they treat.) But moving beyond a random search, I can suggest a number of organizations a caregiver in search of spiritual support might wish to explore.

The Spiritual Care Association (SCA), founded in 1961, was the first multidisciplinary, international organization to dispense evidence-based research updates to spiritual care providers and is now accredited to bestow advanced degrees in multi-faith studies, ministry and chaplaincy, and spiritual care through its University of Theology and Spirituality.[27] The Health Care Chaplaincy Network, another affiliate of SCA, prescribes spiritual-care resources and information to "help people faced with illness and grief find comfort and meaning—whoever they are, whatever they believe, wherever they are."[28]

Community of Hope International, an organization focused on compassionate listening founded in 1994 by Helen Appelberg at St. Luke's Hospital in Houston, presently oversees thirty-six centers in the Episcopal diocese of Texas and eighty-four others in the United States, Canada, Mexico, and Malawi.[29] An even larger organization is Stephen Ministries (its name derives from Ephesians 4:12), which empowers caregivers to extend hope and healing to care receivers by promoting spiritual resources for lay caregivers. Since 1975, Stephen Ministries has trained more than seventy-five thousand spiritual leaders and six hundred thousand volunteers, who serve 1.5 million people who have benefited from one-on-one caring relationships. Stephen Ministries has more than thirteen thousand affiliated congregations representing 180 Christian denominations in the United States, Canada, and thirty other countries.[30]

There is also much to admire in the work of B. J. Miller, who lost both legs and part of an arm in a horrific accident as a Princeton undergraduate and now serves as executive director of the Zen Hospice Project and a palliative care physician at the University of California at San Francisco medical center.[31]

If one belongs to a particular religious denomination, then checking out local synagogues, mosques, and churches may allow one to access congregation-based programs to support informal caregivers.[32] While differing in spiritual beliefs, faith-based institutions that I have visited all foster effective ways of listening to one's inner voices and relating to strangers. Meanwhile, other resources exist to support humanistic, nonreligious, and atheist caregivers.[33]

Novel technological instruments may provide helpful aids in providing care and lessen caregiver stress.[34] AARP, the Alzheimer's Association, and other supportive care groups continually update lists of devices to support caregivers. Telehealth instruments and "nano" technologies facilitate virtual in-home visits. Cameras, robots, and GPS locators not only monitor and track patients' movements, but they also report 911 emergencies.[35]

CONCLUSION

Informal spiritual caregiving is intimate, whether it takes place in hospital rooms or homes. Even with robust access to information and support available to someone like me as a leader in a major medical center, I found caregiving among the most challenging yet rewarding activities I have ever engaged in. Creating and sustaining compassionate caregiving is daunting and involves financial, physical, emotional, social, and spiritual factors. While they are all interconnected, in my life and I believe in the lives of many, the spiritual component is perhaps most central to successful caregiving. In this essay, I have charted some innovations and obstacles to integrating spiritual care into medical delivery. Despite the obstacles I and other caregivers have faced, I believe the prognosis for improved caregiving and in particular spiritual caregiving is positive. Spiritual caregiving has come a long way since the days of Job's questing and Ivan Ilych's suffering, after all.

NOTES

1. Associated Press–NORC Center for Public Affairs Research 2018; Family Caregiver Alliance 2019.
2. Sarton 1973, 21.
3. Accius 2019.
4. Porter 2019.
5. National Alliance for Caregiving and AARP 2020.
6. Verghese 2011.
7. Levine and Reinhard 2016.
8. Eisenberg 2018.
9. Stepler 2015; AARP Public Policy Institute 2015.
10. Roth, Fredman, and Haley 2015.
11. Casarella 2019.
12. Eisenberg 2018.
13. Moore 2010; Topol, Verghese, and Kleinman 2019.
14. Nickell 2015.
15. Roof 1994; Bengston and Silverstein 2019.
16. Moore 2010; Puchalski et al. 2020.
17. Achenbaum and Dyer 2021.
18. Borneman, Ferrell, and Puchalski 2010; Delgado-Guay et al. 2021.
19. Kinghorn 2013.
20. Silva 2013; Pepin and Hebert 2020.
21. Hui et al. 2010; Delgado-Guay et al. 2012; Delgado-Guay et al. 2017.
22. Buck and McMillan 2012; Kelly, May, and Maurer 2016; Vitorino et al. 2017.
23. McMorrow 2018.
24. "Eldercare Locator" n.d.
25. Applebaum, Kulikowski, and Breitbart 2015; Wheeler 2016.
26. Meichenbaum n.d.; Graham 2013.
27. "Spiritual Care Association" 2020.
28. "About Us" 2020.
29. "About COHI" n.d.
30. "History of Stephen Ministries St. Louis" 2020.
31. Rigoglioso 2014.
32. AGIS n.d.
33. Dearie 2018; Radcliffe 2018; Koenig n.d.
34. Wegerer 2019; Sauer 2019; "Family-Caregiver Support" 2020.
35. Mauterstock 2019.

WORKS CITED

AARP Public Policy Institute. 2015. "Caregiving in the U.S." https://www.aarp.org /content/dam/aarp/ppi/2015 /caregiving-in-the-united-states-2015 -report-revised.pdf.
"About COHI." n.d. Community of Hope International. Accessed September 2, 2020. https://www.cohinternational.org /history.
"About Us." 2020. HealthCare Chaplaincy Network. https://www.healthcarechap laincy.org/about-us.html.
Accius, J. C. 2019. "The Evolving Role of Male Family Caregivers." *Aging Today* 40 (5): 5.
Achenbaum, W. A., and C. B. Dyer. 2021. "Mind the Gaps." Archived in the McGovern Medical School, Department of Internal Medicine, Division of Geriatric and Palliative Care, Consortium on Aging.
ACPE, Association of Professional Chaplains, Canadian Association for Spiritual Care, National Association of Catholic Chaplains, and Neshama. 2019. *The Impact of Professional Spiritual Care*. https://indd.adobe.com/view/2d555e8f -5d1a-47bf-ad94-760092053d0b.
AGIS. n.d. "Faith Based Support." Accessed September 2, 2020. http://www.agis .com/eldercare-basics/Support-Services /Faith-Based-Support.
Allen, J. G. 2013. "Hope Is Human." *Bulletin of Menninger Clinic* 77 (4): 302–31.

Ando, M. 2017. "Effects of Music Therapy on the Mood of Family-Caregivers and Care Staffs and Relationships Between Mood and Healing Sense in a Palliative Care Ward." *International Journal of Psychotherapy Practice and Research* 1 (1): 1–6.

Applebaum, A. J., J. R. Kulikowski, and W. Breitbart. 2015. "Meaning-Centered Psychotherapy for Cancer Caregivers." *Palliative and Supportive Care* 13 (6): 1631–41.

Associated Press–NORC Center for Public Affairs Research. 2018. "Long-Term Caregiving: The True Costs of Caring for Aging Adults." https://apnorc.org/wp-content/uploads/2020/02/Long-Term-Caregiving-2018-Report.pdf.

Bengston, V. L., and M. Silverstein, eds. 2019. *Spirituality, Religion, and Aging.* New York: Routledge.

Biggar, A. 2019. "Sacred Singing at the Threshold Between Life and Death." *Aging Today* 40 (3): 1, 15.

Borneman, T., B. Ferrell, and C. M. Puchalski. 2010. "Evaluation of the FICA Tool for Spiritual Assessment." *Journal of Pain and Symptom Management* 40 (2): 163–73.

Buck, H. G., and S. C. McMillan. 2012. "A Psychometric Analysis of the Spiritual Needs Inventory in Informal Caregivers of Patients with Cancer in Hospice Home Care." *Oncology Nursing Forum.* https://works.bepress.com/harleah-buck/9.

"Caregiving." 2020. CancerCare. https://www.cancercare.org/tagged/caregiving.

Casarella, J. 2019. "Caregiving: Stress and Depression." *WebMD.* https://www.webmd.com/anxiety-panic/guide/self-injuring-hurting.

Dearie, J. 2018. "New Parish-Based Program Offers Care to Caregivers." *National Catholic Reporter.* July 5, 2018. https://www.ncronline.org/news/parish/new-parish-based-program-offers-care-caregivers.

Delgado-Guay, M. O., S. McCollom, A. Palma, E. Duarte, M. Grez, and L. Tupper. 2017. "Spirituality Among Latino Caregivers of Patients with Advanced Cancer." *Journal of Clinical Oncology* 35 (31suppl.): 180.

Delgado-Guay, M. O., A. Palma, E. Duarte, M. Grez, L. Tupper, D. D. Lui, and E. Bruera. 2021. "Association Between Spirituality, Religiosity, Spiritual Pain, Symptom Distress, and Quality of Life Among Latin American Patients with Advanced Cancer: A Multicenter Study." *Journal of Palliative Medicine* 24 (11): 1606–15. doi: 10.1089/jpm.2020.0776.

Delgado-Guay, M. O., H. A. Parsons, D. Hui, M. De la Cruz, S. Thorney, and E. Bruera. 2012. "Spirituality, Religiosity, and Spiritual Pain Among Caregivers of Patients with Advanced Cancer." *American Journal of Hospice and Palliative Medicine* 30 (5): 455–61. https://doi.org/10.1177/1049909111458030.

Eisenberg, R. 2018. "The Financial and Personal Toll of Family Caregiving." March 12, 2018. Accessed July 7, 2021. https://www.forbes.com/sites/nextavenue/2018/03/12/the-financial-and-personal-toll-of-family-caregiving/?sh=57e2097a58b8.

"Eldercare Locator." n.d. Accessed September 2, 2020. https://eldercare.acl.gov/Public/Index.aspx.

Evans, A. R., ed. 2011. *Is God Still at the Bedside?* Grand Rapids: Eerdmans.

Family Caregiver Alliance. 2019. "Caregiver Statistics: Demographics." National Center on Caregiving. April 17, 2019. https://www.caregiver.org/caregiver-statistics-demographics.

"Family-Caregiver Support." 2020. Preferred Care at Home. https://preferhome.com/senior-resources/family_caregiver_support.

Graham, J. 2013. "For Traumatized Caregivers, Therapy Helps." *The New Old Age* (blog). *New York Times.* February 22, 2013. https://newoldage.blogs.nytimes.com/2013/02/22/for-traumatized-caregivers-therapy-helps.

"History of Stephen Ministries St. Louis." 2020. Stephen Ministries. https://www.stephenministries.org/aboutus/default.cfm/721?mnblau=1.

Hui, D., M. de la Cruz, S. Thorney, H. A. Parsons, M. O. Delgado-Guay, and E. Bruera. 2010. "The Frequency and

Correlates of Spiritual Distress Among Patients with Advanced Cancer Admitted to an Acute Palliative Care Unit." *American Journal of Hospice and Palliative Care* 28 (4): 264–70. doi: 10 .1177/1049909110385917.

Kelly, J. A., C. S. May, and S. H. Maurer. 2016. "Assessment of the Spiritual Needs of Primary Caregivers of Children with Life-Limiting Illnesses Is Valuable Yet Inconsistently Performed in the Hospital." *Journal of Palliative Medicine* 19 (7): 763–66. doi: 10.1089/jpm.2015.0509.

Kinghorn, W. 2013. "Warren Kinghorn: Asking Broader Questions of Medicine." Faith and Leadership. March 27, 2013. https:// faithandleadership.com/warren -kinghorn-asking-broader-questions -medicine.

Koenig, H. G. n.d. "What Religion Can Do for Your Health." Beliefnet. Accessed September 2, 2020. https://www .beliefnet.com/wellness/health/2006 /05/what-religion-can-do-for-your -health.aspx.

Levine, C., and S. C. Reinhard. 2016. "'It All Falls on Me': Family Caregiver Perspectives on Medication Management, Wound Care, and Video Instruction." *AARP Spotlight* (September 2016): 1–19. https://aarp.org/content/dam/aarp /ppi/2016-08/AARP1078_FamilyCare giver_SpotlightSep6v5.pdf.

Mauterstock, R. 2019. "3 Breakthroughs in Technology to Help Caregivers." *Forbes*, February 1, 2019. https://www.forbes .com/sites/robertmauterstock/2019/02 /01/3-breakthroughs-in-technology-to -help-caregivers/#24656f8ebe6e.

McMorrow, P. 2018. "10 Soul-Healing Tips to Help Prevent Caregiver Burnout." CaringBridge. April 18, 2018. https:// www.caringbridge.org/resources/how -to-avoid-caregiver-burnout.

Meichenbaum, D. n.d. "Self-Care for Trauma Psychotherapists and Caregivers: Individual, Social and Organizational Interventions." Accessed September 2, 2020. https://melissainstitute.org/wp -content/uploads/2016/12/SELF-CARE -FOR-TRAUMA-PSYCHOTHERA

PISTS-AND-CAREGIVERS-changed -26.pdf.

Moore, T. 2010. *Care of Soul in Medicine*. Carlsbad, CA: Hay House.

National Alliance for Caregiving and AARP. 2020. *Caregiving in the U.S. 2020*. https:// www.caregiving.org/wp-content /uploads/2021/01/full-report-caregiving -in-the-united-states-01-21.pdf.

Nickell, C. 2015. *Uniting Faith, Medicine, and Healthcare*. Houston: Institute for Spirituality and Health.

Pepin, E., and J. Hébert. 2020. "Needs of Caregivers of Patients Receiving In-Home Palliative and End-of-Life Care." *Canadian Oncology Nursing Journal* 30 (2): 147–52. doi: 10.5737 /23688076302147152.

Porter, E. 2019. "From Career-Driven to Caregivers." *Houston Chronicle*, September 8, 2019, B5.

Puchalski, C., N. Jafari, H. Buller, T. Haythorn, C. Jacobs, and B. Ferrell. 2020. "Interprofessional Spiritual Care Education Curriculum: A Milestone Toward the Provision of Spiritual Care." *Journal of Palliative Medicine* 23 (6): 777–84.

Radcliffe, S. 2018. "Does Prayer Help or Harm Your Health?" Last modified April 19, 2018. *Healthline News*. https://www .healthline.com/health-news/does -prayer-help-or-harm-your-health#1.

Rigoglioso, M. 2014. "BJ Miller '93: Wounded Healer." *Princeton Alumni Weekly*, February 5, 2014, 37–38.

Roof, W. C. 1994. *A Generation of Seekers*. San Francisco: HarperCollins.

Roth, D. L., L. Fredman, and W. E. Haley. 2015. "Informal Caregiving and Its Impact on Health." *Gerontologist* 55 (2): 309–19. doi: 10.1093/geront/gnu177.

Sarton, M. 1973. *As We Are Now*. New York: W. W. Norton.

Sauer, A. 2019. "7 Technological Innovations for Those with Dementia." *Alzheimers.net* (blog). January 9, 2019. https://www .alzheimers.net/9-22-14-technology-for -dementia.

Silva, A. L., H. J. Teixeira, M. J. Teixeira, and S. Freitas. 2013. "The Needs of Informal Caregivers of Elderly People Living at

Home: An Integrative Review."
Scandinavian Journal of Caring Sciences 27
(4): 792–803. doi: 10.1111/scs.12019.

"Spiritual Care Association." 2020. Spiritual
Care Association. https://spiritualcare
association.org.

Stepler, Renee. 2015. "5 Facts About Family
Caregivers." Pew Research Center.
November 18, 2015. https://www.pew
research.org/fact-tank/2015/11/18/5
-facts-about-family-caregivers.

Topol, E. J., A. Verghese, and A. M. Kleinman.
2019. "Caregiving and the Soul of
Medicine." *Medscape*, November 1, 2019.
https://www.medscape.com/view
article/920514.

Verghese, A. 2011. "Treat the Patient, Not the CT
Scan." *New York Times*, February 26, 2011.
https://www.nytimes.com/2011/02/27
/opinion/27verghese.html.

Vitorino, L. M., L. S. Marins, A. L. G. Lucchetti,
and A. E. O. Santos, J. P. Cruz, P. J. O.
Ortez, and G. Lucchetti. 2018. "Spiritual/
Religious Coping and Depressive

Symptoms in Informal Caregivers of
Hospitalized Older Adults." *Geriatric
Nursing* 39 (1): 48–53. doi: 10.1016/j
.gerinurse.2017.06.001.

Wegerer, J. 2019. "7 Ways Technology Helps
Family Caregivers." A Place for Mom.
March 27, 2019. https://www.aplacefor
mom.com/blog/2013-7-21-technology
-family-caregivers.

Wheeler, E. 2016. "How to Cultivate Self-
Compassion While Caregiving."
Wildflower Center for Emotional
Health. March 18, 2016. https://
wildflowerllc.com/self-compassion
-while-caregiving.

CHAPTER 15

Palliative Care

A Chaplain's Perspective

Bettie Jo Tennon Hightower

Rabbi Alvin Fine encapsulated my decades as a hospital chaplain when he wrote,

> *Birth is a beginning*
> *And death is a destination.*
> *And life is a journey,*
> *A sacred pilgrimage—*
> *To life everlasting.*[1]

Life is fragile. Life is short. It is also a journey, a pilgrimage, to eternal life. I have learned this at countless bedsides.

MINISTRY LEADING TO PALLIATIVE CARE

My work as a chaplain for nearly fifteen years has deep roots in Christian ministry and the medical profession. I served for twelve years in a local United Methodist church and sixteen years as a registered nurse at Houston Methodist Hospital. The move to palliative care, knowing what I know of human flourishing and suffering, waning and waxing, was a natural one.

My entrée to palliative care was intended to allow me to be present to palliative care *staff*, but it soon become clear that I needed to be part of a team in order to provide continuity of care for *patients*. I had served as senior chaplain in intermediate and intensive care, where I learned that a patient's condition could shift hour by hour, minute by waking or sleeping minute. I have also sat on the Biomedical Ethics Committee and the Schwartz Round Committee, from which I learned about complex ethical dilemmas that could evolve into multidisciplinary discussions and recommendations. My transition to the multidisciplinary, intense world of palliative care, therefore, was a natural one. I took a course, Essentials of Palliative Care, from California State University, and I was off and running—or standing, sitting, and kneeling, with an array of not only patients but also families and staff.

THE HEALTH CARE VILLAGE

In my African Native French American heritage, we knew, long before it was popularized, that "it takes a village to raise a child."[2] As a child, all those years ago, in a small remote Texas community, I knew that I was safe even when my parents were absent. This village of adults that cared for us along with our parents included grandparents, aunts, uncles, play uncles, and play aunts.[3] In the same way, health care professionals are a community of caring, compassionate, dedicated individuals whose life-giving, life-sustaining health care education, credentials, and experiences constitute a village created to provide health and healing to those who come for care.

Yet, despite all of the training, health care professionals are aware that disease, suffering, and pain are constantly challenging the latest training and technology. Change in the condition of a patient can be inevitable. When this change occurs, we are called to continue helping our patients. Patients die in our care, much to the dismay and distress of all involved, most notably the patient's family and health care professionals. This is not, however, the time for palliative care to begin.

Palliative care starts at the *beginning* of any illness. Palliation is always a part of the healing process. Figure 15.1 demonstrates what palliative care looks like at the beginning of an illness, when most of the care is curative or primary in nature, with a smaller portion of the care devoted to spiritual and emotional dimensions. Again, palliative care starts at the beginning of illness—not just in its final stages, when death is imminent.

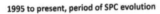

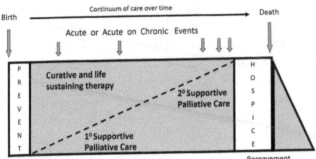

FIG. 15.1 Palliative care across the care and time continuum. Created by Robert L. Fine, MD, FACP, FAAHPM, Director—Office of Clinical Ethics and Palliative Care, Baylor Scott and White Health (2015) and used with permission of Baylor Scott & White Health Office of Clinical Ethics and Palliative Care.

This diagram illustrates that acute events tend to come closer in time as the end of life approaches. Further illustrated is that there is a role for both primary care and specialty palliative care *throughout* the patient care process. They can exist together. Both are essential to the long-term care of a patient in the midst of life's fragility. Palliative care can be minimal at the beginning— perhaps management of symptoms such as pain or nausea or vomiting—but its role can increase as the illness takes a direction other than curative. With palliative care as part of the management of health from the start of an illness, the patient's values, wishes, desires, spirituality, and mental health are part of the healing process from start to finish. Plan-of-care discussions become a normal part of the process. Bereavement care is begun before death.

Ideally, I think, palliative care can work in tandem with primary or curative care. Too often, however, due to strained resources and traditional concep- tions of medical care, palliative care begins only when curative care is deemed no longer viable. My preference, as a chaplain, is to have palliative care pro- fessionals as part of the team earlier than they currently are in practice. Yet the discipline is young at this time, and that integration, I believe, will occur as the value of palliative care is increasingly acknowledged within the med- ical community. Perhaps in the future an advance care planning guide and consultation, which enables the patient to begin talking with family mem- bers and physicians about what they would like to happen for the course of their care, will become integral rather than optional in patient care.

THE CHAPLAIN STEPS IN

When a patient enters the hospital, what I call a patient's medical story becomes pivotal. Their world changes significantly. They learn a new language. They learn a new diagnosis. The very source of their being undergoes an intense stretching into the unknown world of health care. As a nurse, I learned that a patient's life becomes a world of ups and downs, gains and losses, around physical well-being and healing. These are moments for a patient of life and death. Life as they once knew it is threatened, and what they anticipate they do with a sense of dread.[4] In this context, what Rodney Tucker, director of the University of Alabama Center for Palliative and Supportive Care, calls the five F's help a patient and family make decisions about health care:[5] fear, family and friends, faith, finances, and facts. The *facts* of the disease they learn from health care practitioners, who are accustomed to explaining in much detail, candor, and compassion. Yet facts are just part of the medical story. There are *financial* decisions to be made. "Will my family be able to pay our bills if I am laid up sick?" There is the inevitability of *fear.* "Will I live to make it through this disease? And if I do live, what will life be like? What will happen to my *family and friends,* if I die?" Then there is the aspect of *faith.* In the South, where I serve, a patient and family's faith often rises to the top of decision-making, especially as end of life approaches. Faith does not always simplify decisions; it often complicates them.

Into that complexity steps the chaplain. The chaplain's role in the healing process is to attend to the patient's inner life. This is the life story that patients bring with them: the legends, the tragedies, the joys, the dreams, the hopes, the values, and the resources the patient brings to the health care setting. As a nurse, I was in the operating room. The surgeon knew the physical landscape of the patient's anatomy and physiology. Analogously, the chaplain is trained to become familiar with the more amorphous world that makes up the spiritual anatomy of the patient.

For patients, this life story, whether known fully or unknown at the time, begins to shape the decisions made about health care. The tragedies they remember come to life and guide how they will view the medical story and the rest of their lives. All of the experiences they have in life, as well as those things and persons they hold valuable, shape their decisions. The dreams they have held for retirement or of seeing their children go to college or of becoming grandparents—all values are brought to bear on this time in their lives.

For the chaplain, a patient is not the gallbladder in Room 488B or the heart transplant in Room 692C. Patients have a life story that accompanies them to the hospital, like an overnight bag or suitcase. Their life story influences how they receive information on their diagnoses, how they determine their course of action, and how they shape whether they will choose to live or die. The five Fs are especially important. Patients turn first to their family and friends, then to their faith, then to their fear, then to their finances, and finally to the facts of their illness. From this they weave an integrated narrative that lends itself to living a life of integrity, no matter the length of their lives.

At this point, the chaplain comes alongside as an *anamcara*, as a *soul friend*.[6] As a soul friend, the chaplain is available to assist in the patient's quest for meaning during hospitalization and afterward. The chaplain can help the patient discover spiritual pain, such as the need for meaning in life and illness. Additionally, the chaplain can help the patient discern a need for forgiveness and relational healing, to name but a few of the weighty matters that surface during illness.

FOUR MODES OF PASTORAL CARE

To help with the morass of competing sensibilities, many chaplains have turned to a book by William A. Clebsch and Charles R. Jaekle, *Pastoral Care in Historic Perspective*.[7] Clebsch and Jaekle's work describes four modes of pastoral care: healing, sustaining, guiding, and reconciling. These four modes circumscribe the ministry of the chaplain. Initially introduced to me twenty years ago, around the early 1990s, they have proven instrumental in the ways I as a chaplain would like to see my ministry develop: helping patients access their hopes and dreams as they lean into the legends, the tragedies, the experiences, and the values that they call upon in order to make life decisions.

The Healing Mode of Pastoral Care

Chaplains are adept at the healing of things that have been pushed aside or failed to surface in the normal course of life. For instance, I was making rounds on about a half dozen palliative care patients at the end of the day. I wanted to be sure that everyone who desired one would have a pastoral visit before a long weekend. Upon my entering the room of a more than ninety-year-old female patient, she began to offer me a life review. She told me that she had lived a good life. She told me about how she enjoyed driving herself to her favorite hamburger place with her friend, who did not drive. She named a few nearby eateries that she enjoyed. It was on one of those trips, she told me, when she went to get a hamburger and milkshake, that she became ill. She was alone on the trip this time. When she became short of breath, a man stopped what he was doing and helped her. He took responsibility for getting her to the hospital. She was grateful for this kind man who had been so sensitive and caring to her in her time of need. She said that she had been told previously by leading physicians that these episodes of shortness of breath would continue to come. She had been told, too, that surgery was too risky for her and thus was not advisable. At that point in the story, she said, "You know, I don't know what happened to my hamburger and milkshake." At this, she chuckled. I chuckled with her (humor can be healing). She talked about how she thought her children would stop her from driving herself. She said that she would not be happy about that, but she would comply if they thought that was the best. She talked more of her good life as the wife of a physician, now deceased. She talked. I listened. I coached her in telling her life story, and I offered her a blessing. I laughed with her about her stories. I even gave her some humor back. Because she was being discharged that evening, and because she mentioned that she didn't remember what happened to her hamburger and shake, in my parting with her, I told her that the only thing I was worried about was when she would get her hamburger. She let out a hearty laugh. During our forty-five minutes or so together, she told me, "I am glad you came today. You are probably the last pastor I will talk to, that I tell my story to." She said, "I don't know how it is that God sent you by here today, but I am glad you came."

I truly believe that I became her confessor that day, the one to whom she bared her soul. This was her life story. This was her confession. I cannot help but believe that somehow some spiritual and emotional "healing" in that happenstance (though more planned than she realized) visit far outweighed the physical healing that leading physicians had already told her would not take place on this side of eternity.

The Sustaining Mode of Pastoral Care

Sometimes illness is such that the patient has to learn to live with chronic, debilitating disease. Sometimes there is the need to envision a new normal that allows assimilation of the illness in their lives.

I met a young man in his thirties in the intensive care unit. The first time I met him, he was weeping, lying in bed, feeling distraught. He shared his life story of heartache. He was a diabetic. He had lost his sight. He had lost his job. He had lost his home. Finally, he had lost his wife. He wept the whole time we were together. I listened. I offered prayer at the end of our visit. He appeared a bit more peaceful when I left.

The next time I saw him, he was in a regular medical bed. He was in "child's pose" on his bed. It was not the restful yoga child's pose. It was with his face buried in the bed, weeping like a child with his rear end in the air. As he continued to weep, I listened and then began to console him with scripture. In my own faith tradition as a Judeo-Christian, I believe that God has a plan for our welfare and not for harm for all of us, to give us a future with hope. I had identified earlier that he was a Christian, and so I began reminding him of the promises of God. The nurse came in to give him medications. He had been refusing his medications and his food, I was told. At this point, his crying began to subside.

I realized that I had offered words of hope from scripture on both visits. I had listened to his distress on both visits. I had consoled him on previous visits. I had returned to visit him and to be present with him. Still, I felt, for his own good, that a more direct approach might be helpful to him. As the mother of two sons, I took a different approach. I asked him, "Are you able to sit up?" He responded that he could. Gently, I coaxed him further, "Then what would happen if you sat up and took the medications the nurse has for you?" Without a word, he sat on the side of the bed and took his medications. Pressing a bit further, I asked him, "What would happen if you ate the food on your tray to help you get better?" He moved from the side of the bed to the chair with the food tray in front of him. I then sat silently with him for about five to seven more minutes. I was remembering how Job's friends in the Bible sat with him for seven days before saying anything. Then I got up, thanked him for allowing me to visit him, and told him that I would return the next day to see how he was doing. I told him that in the meantime we had chaplains available twenty-four hours a day, if he felt as if he needed to talk some more. I went back the next day; he was sitting up in a chair, eating his food. He was discharged from the hospital the following day.

Sometimes, in the midst of life, mystery happens. I don't know today, what, if anything, I said or did to make a difference in this young man's life. I believe that, in the silence, the listening, the encouragement, and the hearing of scripture, perhaps mystery did happen for this young man. And I hope he is living the promises of God today.

The Guiding Mode of Pastoral Care

Guiding helps patients and their family to receive help or direction, which they may not even be aware of needing at the time. This is one mode with which I tend to be less direct. I believe that patients have the answers needed for their care. Sometimes a bit of insight or appropriate questions help them to become aware of their own internal resources, resilience, and self-knowledge.

Early one morning I came to the intensive care unit and was greeted by the nurses saying, "Get the priest . . . get the priest." A patient had just died. Her two daughters had been with her throughout her hospitalization. Her son had just arrived from Mexico. From the room, I heard the bitterest weeping I have ever heard. It was the deep weeping I imagine when I read the words of Jesus in the Bible, that "there will be great weeping and gnashing of teeth." The patient and her family were Spanish-speaking and from Mexico. I do not know why, even today, but I instinctually checked the chart before calling the priest. It might have been all those years in nursing quality assurance, when I reviewed charts for the physicians on a daily basis, that caused me to check the chart. It might have been the awareness of the shortage of priests and the need to make an appropriate assessment before calling for a priest. Or it may be a chaplain's instinct. It turns out that the patient was not Catholic at all. She and her family were Jewish.

I called the Texas Medical Center Jewish chaplain. I told her what was happening and described the state of the patient's son. This dear sister in ministry said the magical words that I wished to hear but was reluctant to express. She said, "Do you want me to come?" Since the patient was from Mexico, and consistent with her faith, the family's major concern was to to expedite care so that she could be buried as soon as possible. The global services department was able to help with getting the body back to Mexico through appropriate international channels. With all of these matters being cared for, something unusual happened when the Jewish chaplain arrived. With logistical matters resolved, thanks to global services, the chaplain's role took priority. The Jewish chaplain asked the patient's son if he'd like her to begin the Mourner's Kaddish. This simple act seemed to ground the son in his faith. The chaplain provided the son with a yarmulke. Then the patient's son began praying, and his tears for a period of time dried.

I believe that the chaplain and I both participated in guiding this family, who were, to use Judeo-Christian imagery, *in a foreign land*. They had come in hopes of a cure, which they did not receive in the way they wished. But with the chaplain, they were able to get back to their roots, to their family heritage. Guidance took place, although physical healing did not take place, in this foreign land, which had offered so much promise and hope for physical healing.

The Reconciling Mode of Pastoral Care

Reconciliation is making peace with the past that we have been at odds with—a person, an institution, a circumstance, or a situation that happened in our lives. It is a coming to terms with things as they are and not as we would want them to be.

As we worked hard to save the life of a forty-one-year-old Muslim man with a young wife and two sons, we knew that the time of his death was near. During remission, the patient had made his pilgrimage to Mecca. He was now back in the hospital. I called for an imam, who had volunteered his services to the hospital. Since it was just before Ramadan, the imam told me that he would be at the hospital by late in the evening or by noon the next day. As I waited with the family, I saw what I could tell was a holy man. I had never met the imam, but I knew inwardly it was he. He came sooner than he had said he would. As we talked afterward, he shared that he had read the Quran and prayed with the patient and his family. I will never forget how he told me that one of his prayers is always "Allah, if it is good for me to live, let me live; if it is good for me to die, let me die." In essence, the imam offered reconciliation with a different future without this patient but with the conviction that Allah was in charge.

CONCLUSION

During my three decades in health care and a decade and a half as a chaplain, I have kept in mind the life of Maimonides,[8] a medieval Jewish physician, philosopher, and Torah scholar, who claimed that the Eternal Providence appointed him to watch over the life and health of God's creatures. This conception of care is relevant for all health care providers. We are involved in *holy work, holy life*—the work, the life, I believe, to which all of us in the patient's village are called to participate. From a friend and chaplain in another institution in the Texas Medical Center, I learned this meditation, which provides an apt closing to this essay on various modes of care. "May we all . . . experience deepest well-being, happiness, health, and freedom from suffering!" The *we* in this prayer does not include patients only but also caregivers of all stripes everywhere, trained and untrained, dispassionate and the passionately devoted. All of us have life stories, which give us the opportunity to experience deepest well-being in the villages, global and local, we occupy and help shape.

NOTES

1. Quoted in Roscher 2013.
2. Stefano 2012.
3. "Play" aunts, uncles, cousins, grandmothers, and grandfathers are endearing terms used in African-descent communities to represent any adults or others who are particularly special to a child although often unrelated biologically to the child.
4. Lester 1995, 35.
5. Tucker 2017.
6. Groves and Klauser 2009.
7. Clebsch and Jaekle 1964.
8. Seeskin 2017.

WORKS CITED

Clebsch, W. A., and C. R. Jaekle. 1964. *Pastoral Care in Historic Perspective*. New York: Jason Aronson.

Groves, R. F., and H. A. Klauser. 2009. *The American Book of Living and Dying: Lessons in Healing Spiritual Pain*. Berkeley: Celestial Arts.

Lester, A. D. 1995. *Hope in Pastoral Care and Counseling*. Louisville: Westminster John Knox.

Lynn, J. 2005. "Living Long in Fragile Health: The New Demographics Shape End of Life Care." In *Improving End of Life Care: Why Has It Been So Difficult?*, edited by B. Jennings, G. E. Kaebnick, and T. H. Murray, S14–S18. Garrison, NY: Hastings Center.

Roscher, E. 2013. "The Sacred Pilgrimage." *Keeping Faith Today* (blog). October 2, 2013. https://keepingfaithtoday.com/2013/10/02/the-sacred-pilgrimage.

Seeskin, K. 2017. "Maimonides." In *The Stanford Encyclopedia of Philosophy*. Spring 2017 ed. Edited by E. N. Zalta. https://plato.stanford.edu/entries/maimonides.

Stefano, D. 2012. "What 'It Takes a Village to Raise a Child' Really Means." *HuffPost*. Last updated April 28, 2012. https://www.huffpost.com/entry/what-it-takes-a-village-t_b_1304689.

Tucker, R. O. 2017. "Can Virtual Palliative Care Consultations Be Successful?" Interview by T. Lee. *NEJM Catalyst*. July 10, 2017. https://catalyst.nejm.org/virtual-palliative-care-consultations.

CHAPTER 16

Lucia's Dream

A Holistic Approach to Adolescents with Cancer

Tullio Proserpio, Elena Pagani Bagliacca,
Giovanna Sironi, and Andrea Ferrari

VERONICA AND HER CAREGIVERS

Veronica was a seventeen-year-old with sarcoma of the skull base. While receiving treatment she had bonded well with the medical team and especially with the chaplain. She had regular meetings with him right from the start, even when her chances of cure still seemed to be good. When her disease relapsed and proved unresponsive to further therapy, Veronica asked to be told all about it in detail. She was confused at first ("*Why do they keep giving me treatments but I always get worse?*"), then angry ("*I can't believe there's no cure for me!*") and afraid ("*I don't want to die!*"). With the support of her family and a concerted effort on the part of the whole health care team, she came to accept her fate. She asked the chaplain, "*What do you think will happen to me after I die? What happens when your eyes close for the last time?*" One evening, well aware of her imminent death, Veronica showed remarkable lucidity and courage when she asked all the doctors on the ward to come to her bedside and thanked them for all their efforts. "*Thank you anyways,*" she said, "*even if you haven't been successful. You're the best doctors in the world. I know you've done everything you could.*" It was Veronica who comforted the medical team. She could see the powerlessness of defeat in their eyes and the emotional difficulty of facing a young girl who knew she was dying. "*I'm fine, doctor, seriously. Don't pull that face.*" Turning to the chaplain, who had spoken to her not long before, Veronica added, "*I die with a smile, thinking of the pope's smile.*"

We learn a great deal about holistic health care from Veronica. We learn that she has a young but vibrant spirituality. We learn about the indispensability of spiritual companions, such as chaplains. We learn about hope. We learn about the power of illusion. We learn a great deal just by listening to a young woman who would not even celebrate her eighteenth birthday.

A PLACE FOR ADOLESCENTS WITH CANCER

In recent decades, the scientific community has started to acknowledge that adolescents with cancer form a group of patients with unique characteristics. They inhabit what could be called a no-man's-land between pediatric and adult services.[1] The peculiar characteristics of this age group are various: a distinctive cancer type distribution and tumor biology, or the lower utilization of referral cancer services and low participation in clinical trials (which is considered one of the main causes of worse survival probabilities for adolescent patients when compared with children affected by the same pathologies, at least when taking in consideration leukemia, medulloblastoma, soft-tissue sarcoma, and bone sarcoma). Among the other unique needs of this population, it is important to consider their psychosocial needs, which often are inadequately addressed.[2] Adolescence is a period during which an individual's personality and identity evolve and develop, gaining their independence. The diagnosis of a tumor, the therapies, and their adverse effects represent a complex trauma that is not simple to manage for young patients. Dealing with the establishment of a sense of identity, exploring sexuality (closely related to self-esteem, which, in turn, is affected by body image), evolving interpersonal relationships, and making decisions about education and employment are affected by a diagnosis of malignant disease and embarking on treatment. The adverse effects of therapy alone are sufficient to derail the normal process of maturation in adolescents, and developmental regression is common.

A multidisciplinary approach to the care of adolescents with cancer needs to take into account all of the complex psychological needs of these patients. This is not simple, since adolescents occupy the middle ground between children and older adults: experience tells us that neither the classic pediatric approach nor the adult model of care is ideally suited to meet the needs of these special patients. Although developing a dedicated model of care for adolescents is not simple, it is obvious that the approach should be age-specific, with some key points to keep in mind. Among these, a special attention to psychological support, based on the concept of maintaining patients' normalcy, enabling them to continue living their lives as normally as possible, is essential.

For these reasons, at the Pediatric Oncology Unit of the Istituto Nazionale dei Tumori in Milan we developed the Youth Project, dedicated to teenagers and young adults.[3] The primary goals of this program are three: (1) to optimize clinical aspects (i.e., patients' inclusion in clinical trials, psychosocial support, fertility-preserving facilities, and access to care after completing cancer therapy), (2) to promote patients' normalcy by providing age-specific spaces (well-equipped multifunctional rooms, a classroom, a gym), and (3) to develop special dedicated activity projects.

The model of care of the Youth Project has some unique aspects: three specialists in clinical psychology are permanent members of the staff, and one of them is specifically dedicated to adolescents and young adult patients to guarantee a psychosocial support. The psychological team actively collaborates with the spiritual assistant (a daily presence at the unit), educators (one of whom is dedicated to adolescents), social workers, and teachers (one high school teacher). Moreover, within the pediatric unit, we have organized a multifunctional room dedicated exclusively to adolescents for socializing, recreation, and activities, with TV, couches, some computers with internet connections, musical instruments, and a library with books, magazines, and DVDs. The costs of establishing the project are covered by private funds (Associazione Bianca Garavaglia onlus), without incurring additional public expense.

The distinctive characteristic of the project is that of organizing artistic projects aimed at giving voice to adolescent patients, giving them the opportunity to tell their stories and enabling the medical staff to gain a different view of their inner world.[4] These support projects include creative laboratories designed to occupy patients for several months (see table 16.1), which are organized differently over a long period.

Creative activities, in which art is used as the principal means of expression, are run by experts, who work together with an educator. This solution has proven successful in helping patients feel part of a group, cope better with their disease, and feel special. These projects should also be seen as a complement to the medical and psychological activities undertaken to sustain the continuity of patients' lives. Through these activities, patients find a way to

Table 16.1   Creative and artistic projects of the Youth Project, developed over the years, with teenagers' words

Publication	Brief description of the project	Patients' voices
L. Veneroni et al., *Tumori* 101, no. 6 (2015): 626–30	Twenty-four patients (from fifteen to twenty years) took part in the project (from April to December 2012); they designed their own fashion collection in all its various stages under the artistic direction of a well-known fashion designer.	Valeria (fifteen years, affected by soft-tissue sarcoma): "This was a creative way to go beyond the limits that have been imposed on us by the doctors and our parents. We created something beautiful, and not only for ourselves but for others too." Federica (sixteen years, bone sarcomas): "I realized that I didn't need to feel ashamed of having no hair, that I didn't need to be afraid of looking at myself in the mirror. I realized that I look good even like this."
A. Ferrari et al., *Journal of Clinical Oncology* 33, no. 2 (2015): 218–21	With help from famous Italian singers, twenty patients (from fifteen to twenty-five years) told their story in music, writing a song called "Nuvole di ossigeno" (Clouds of oxygen). The project took eight months to complete. The video of the song can be found on YouTube: https://youtube.com/watch?v=9Ji-lOMI9zU.	"The best feeling of all is knowing you have a future and that it's in your hands." "But I need to feel that you're on my side, here with me." "Take me away, let's get away from here, please, take me to another world."
A. Ferrari et al., *Journal of Clinical Oncology* 35, no. 19 (2017): 2209–12	From autumn 2015 to summer 2016, thirty adolescent and young adult cancer patients took part in a photography project called "Searching for Happiness."	Lorenzo (treated for ependymoma) took pictures from unusual perspectives and explained, "My photographs are the metaphor of how I try to deal with the obstacles that life places before me and how I seek happiness. I have learned how to try to overcome the obstacles from my worst limitation, the visual impairment caused by my disease. . . . Maybe the important thing is not to see the whole picture but to look (and live) from as many alternative and original viewpoints as possible."

Publication	Brief description of the project	Patients' voices
P. Gaggiotti et al., *Tumori* 105, no. 3 (2019): 193–98	Twenty patients (from fifteen to twenty-six years) participated in a project revolving around the question "What shall I do when I grow up?" They wrote a brief account of what they hoped to do as adults. Using theatrical costumes, they then dressed up in their chosen role for a photo shoot with a well-known professional photographer.	Camilla, twenty-six years old, dressed as a genie in a lamp: "I love people, and I especially love making them happy, making them smile and laugh, surprising them, giving them courage. I like taking part in making dreams happen, finding solutions to put into practice in the world that will change this society." Lucy, eighteen years old, dressed as a soft toy tamer: "I love being with children, so I think as a grownup I'd probably enjoy being a soft toy trainer or tamer. It's important for our cuddly toys to be able to cope with all kinds of adventure alongside the child they belong to."
A. Ferrari et al., *Tumori* 103, no. 2 (2017): e9–e14; A. Ferrari et al, *Pediatric Blood and Cancer* 64, no. 9 (2017), doi: 10.1002/pbc.26516	From May to October 2016, twenty-nine young people (from fifteen to twenty-five years old) worked on a Christmas song. The video of the song, titled "Palle di Natale" (Christmas balls) (https://www.youtube.com/watch?v=hFNXCuPCb1A), went viral, with more than fourteen million views.	"The real normal is the shape we give things," sings Samuele. "It is up to us, the patients, to decide what Christmas means to us, and how we want to experience it. . . . Christmas together with those who're left, here at my side, in spirit, our star lighting our way. You'll be my answer, I'll start again, become stronger." This is an explicit reference to the traveling companions who have been lost.
A. Ferrari et al., *Journal of Medical Humanities* (2019), doi: 10.1007/s10912-019-09561-1	Nineteen patients (from fifteen to twenty-five years) participated in a four-month project to develop a graphic novel, a story about superheroes. The title chosen by the teens was "Loop: Indietro non si torna" (Loop: There's no going back), describing their aim to keep looking ahead, one way or another. Patients created their own characters, bringing out the superhero inside them, and succeeded in voicing their dreams and fears.	Synapse: "I would have liked to get up and run away, but there is no way to escape from myself." Electra feels "the earth growl and swallow everything up in a sepulchral silence, like a sudden annihilating storm." Luke tells of his "fear of finding no friends who can help him grow up." Alex describes a recurrent nightmare in which he "falls and is impaled on the sharp tips of the rocks."

Table 16.1 Creative and artistic projects of the Youth Project, developed over the years, with teenagers' words (*continued*)

Publication	Brief description of the project	Patients' voices
S. Signoroni et al., *Pediatric Blood and Cancer* 66, no. 5 (2019): e27630	The *Sei tu l'estate* (La danza della pioggia al contrario) (Summer is you [Rain dance in reverse]) music project involved forty-five patients (from fifteen to twenty-six years old). With professional help, the patients wrote music and lyrics, sang their song, and recorded a video clip: https://youtu.be/Q5FSCMUVg0E. Patients wanted to focus on their longing for summer, traveling, dreaming, and dancing and to bring that energy into the hospital.	"I'll smile despite the rain, because summer is you, if you dance with me, dance, and don't worry anymore." "We'll travel at night so that when you ask me where we're going, I can promise there'll be sunshine." "You've hidden your happiness under the sand, in that spot on the beach that you whispered to me."
L. Veneroni et al., *Tumori* 105, no. 6 (2019): 529–30. doi: 10.1177/03008 91618805655	First individual project of the Youth Project: a book written by Leo, an adolescent amputated for a femoral osteosarcoma, entitled "Dal Settimo cielo al Settimo piano" (From the seventh floor to seventh heaven).	"I learned in my years spent motorcycling. My motto was: Put your head down, but never lower your gaze—and it still is. As my trainer used to say, anyone can ride fast down a straight road, but it's on the bends that you have to step on the gas. Now I'm in a race full of bends, but it's the most important circuit of my life, and I have to overcome my fears and win."

express unvoiced feelings, process their thoughts, and integrate the negative experience of the disease in their personality.[5]

SPIRITUALITY IN ADOLESCENTS

As we have mentioned, cancer patients may have special needs that often go unnoticed. Today it is obvious that managing these additional needs has become an increasingly important goal of care providers. In particular, adequate management of the psychological and social issues of patients in their teen years is essential because they experience disease at a time when they are undergoing major emotional and physical changes.[6] In the complex psychological and social sphere of teenagers with cancer, spirituality also has an important place. It is characteristic of adolescents to wonder about the meaning of life and what the future holds in store. For such reasons, care of adolescents with cancer around the globe should consider also young patients' *spiritual* needs.

Everyone, of course, has spiritual needs, and some have religious needs. The importance of spirituality is highlighted in a document from the US National Cancer Institute, available at http://www.cancer.gov/cancertopics /pdq/supportivecare/spirituality/HealthProfessional/page2. This document states that

> specific religious beliefs and practices should be distinguished from the idea of a universal capacity for spiritual and religious experiences. This distinction is important conceptually for understanding various aspects of evaluation and the role of different beliefs, practices, and experiences in coping with cancer. The most useful general distinction to make in this context is between religion and spirituality. There is no general agreement on definitions of either term, but there is general agreement on the usefulness of this distinction. (https://www.ncbi .nlm.nih.gov/books/NBK66000) Religion can be viewed as a specific set of beliefs and practices associated with a recognized religion or denomination. Spirituality is generally recognized as encompassing experiential aspects, whether related to engaging in religious practices or to acknowledging a general sense of peace and connectedness. Some individuals consider themselves both spiritual and religious; some

may consider themselves religious but not spiritual. Others, including some atheists and agnostics, may consider themselves spiritual but not religious.[7]

For some parents, spirituality has facilitated transcendent meanings and hope; for some, spirituality has offered personal strength, solace, guidance, and meaning-making; and for several parents, spirituality has buffered personal isolation through supportive relationships within their faith community.[8] Even teenagers recognize, in their depth, the true existential questions: Why am I alive? What is the meaning of my life? During adolescence, in fact, individuals tend to distance themselves from their parents and their parents' beliefs and teachings; they therefore tend to change their search for the meaning of life, or, in other words, their approach to spirituality.

CHIARA AND HER CHAPLAIN

Chiara, a sixteen-year-old with osteosarcoma, in further progression after various courses of chemotherapy and surgeries, one day mustered the courage to talk with the chaplain about her fear of dying, something she had never previously had the strength to mention to anyone else, not even her parents or her best friend. *"I'm scared of dying. It's not fair. I'm young,"* she told the chaplain. Then she asked, *"Are there lots of patients who tell you that?"* The chaplain answered, *"No, not many, which goes to show how brave you are. Being afraid of dying is normal, you know."* Chiara and the chaplain had several meetings, often discussing the topic of death. The priest never tried to convince Chiara to believe in God or heaven, but he was always willing to listen to her as she voiced her doubts. He explained his idea of faith—but also how cancer (and the terminal stages of the disease) can be experienced with or without faith. Having the chance to talk about it helped the girl to go toward her death with a greater degree of serenity.

The chaplain plays an essential role in holistic health care. Within the Milan Youth Project, the dedicated multidisciplinary team of professionals includes a chaplain. This is a Catholic priest with specific training, in our case, a graduate of the Psychology Institute at the Pontificia Università Gregoriana in Rome who holds a doctorate in pastoral health at the Pontificia Università Lateranense. Since 2011, the activities of a chaplain have been reorganized and better structured, and this figure is now acknowledged as a permanent member of staff. Some of the chaplain's time is spent on religious procedures, such as celebrating Mass, giving blessings, saying prayers, administering the sacraments (sacrament of the sick, baptism, reconciliation, Eucharist, and confirmation) at the request of patients and families; he is also involved in organizing religious experiences (such as pilgrimages) and cooperating with local religious communities.[9] In addition to these general practices, the chaplain's work includes

- daily visits to the ward and the outpatient clinic or day hospital
- daily meetings with the psychologists on staff
- biweekly meetings with doctors and/or nurses

Daily talks with patients, relatives, and staff members enable the chaplain to assess the spiritual needs of patients and their relatives. These talks allow chaplains to identify special cases that warrant particular attention and counseling and to discuss the management of cases. A typical scenario involves the chaplain providing support for terminal patients and their families, including individual support during the process of grief. This spiritual support is not only offered at the end of a patient's life; it is also available as a resource throughout the period of patient care.[10] Pastoral counseling and spiritual support are also offered to non-Catholic patients and families. For non-Catholic believers, the chaplain contacts a local representative for their particular religious affiliation. The topic of spiritual needs is generally also discussed with nonbelieving families. The chaplain also periodically attends meetings and events organized for and by adolescents involved in the Youth Project.[11]

In 2014, we published a first study that described a series of patients referred for psychological consultation and for spiritual assistance, focusing on new cases diagnosed between January and December 2012. Our chaplain provided specific support to two children (eleven and twelve years old) and twenty adolescents (fifteen to nineteen years old) and young adults (twenty to twenty-four years old). Spiritual assistance was also provided to twenty-nine parents of children and nine parents of older patients. Table 16.2 reports the reasons why adolescent patients had talks with the chaplain.[12]

In many cases, patients asked the chaplain about the meaning of their illness: *"Why me? Why now? What did I do wrong?"* Sometimes patients asked

TABLE 16.2 Reasons for adolescent patients requesting spiritual support

Reasons to request spiritual support	No. of patients
The meaning of illness	6
Dejection due to persistent dependence on parents	5
Issues relating to patients' religious communities	5
Sense of guilt for mistreating parents	2
Doubts about the existence of God	2
Concerns about death	2

the chaplain for advice because they felt the burden of still having to depend on their parents ("*I was just beginning to become independent. I was pleased to grow up and start to take care of myself. . . . Now I feel forced to depend on my parents again, and this makes me angry*"). In some cases, patients needed to talk to the chaplain about their religious doubts ("*If God exists, why did he let me become ill?*") or their concerns about death. It is noteworthy that the reasons for requesting spiritual support only partially overlap with the motives behind requests to see a psychologist; of course, a commonality exists, but this is a further reason to underline the need for cooperation between the psychology team and the spiritual assistant. Our clinical experience shows that young patients found the figure of the chaplain less "formal" than those of the psychologists, and so he was seen as "someone easy to talk to." However, it is important to note that psychologists and spiritual assistants may approach the same so-called problem in two different ways, which may be complementary and not redundant—for example, the meaning of illness, dejection due to persistent dependence on parents, or concerns about death. A crucial point is that an effective relationship between the spiritual assistant (in our context represented by the chaplain) and young patients is critical to provide true spiritual support and can be achieved only with the daily presence and involvement of the counselor from the beginning of the treatment pathway. Meeting the spiritual assistant every day, as a member of the multidisciplinary team, makes it easier for patients and families to accept the help he or she can offer.

Following the study previously discussed, we carried out a survey in pediatric oncology centers in Italy and Spain to examine the situation concerning the provision of spiritual support in pediatric oncology centers, with a special focus on adolescents.[13] An ad hoc questionnaire was distributed, including multiple-choice questions on whether or not spiritual support was available, the spiritual counselor's role, how often the spiritual counselor visited the unit, and the type of training this person had received, regardless of his or her being a chaplain or any another spiritual figure in the different centers involved in the survey.

This study told us that the role of the spiritual counselor within the pediatric oncology scenario was neither adequate nor standardized. Although the survey showed that a spiritual support service was available at twenty-four of the twenty-six responding centers in Italy and thirty-four of thirty-six in Spain, some critical aspects emerged. First, the training received by the spiritual counselor was exclusively theological in most cases, with medical or psychological training in merely a few cases. Second, in both countries, the spiritual counselor was mainly involved in providing religious services and support at the terminal stage of the disease. Cooperation of the spiritual counselors with caregivers was reported as only 27.3 percent and 46.7 percent of the Italian and Spanish centers, respectively, while the *daily* presence of the chaplain on the ward was even less: 18.2 percent and 26.7 percent.

We have recently published another study aiming to describe the demand for spiritual counseling among adolescents treated at our center. The study reports that in the period from January 1, 2016, to December 31, 2017, thirty-three adolescent and young adult (aged fifteen to twenty-four years) patients had from two to twelve (median four) one-to-one talks with the chaplain.

The talk with the chaplain was not systematically proposed to all adolescent patients. The referral of cases to the chaplain may follow three different paths:

- The clinical staff (doctors or nurses) or the psychology team of the unit report to the chaplain those specific cases that may necessitate particular attention and counseling.
- The chaplain comes into direct contact with the patient during daily visits to the ward and initiates a relationship.
- The patient specifically requests a talk with the chaplain. Some of those conversations—in the patients' own words—were good examples of the spiritual needs of young people and how it is important to support these needs.

However the relationship between the chaplain and the adolescent develops, it is not an ancillary relationship. It is fundamental to helping adolescents deal with cancer while living and dying. Think again of Chiara, whose relationship with the chaplain was built on enough trust that she would talk honestly in ways that she would not even with her family and friends. The chaplain can provide that safe space where an adolescent with cancer can explore anything, including perhaps her or his nascent spirituality.

THE POWER OF ILLUSION

Recent research has demonstrated that spiritual or religious practices are resources that can help patients cope better with disease and suffering.[14] A correlation between hope and quality of life has been reported, and hope has been included among the aspects of quality of life measured in patients with various neoplasms.[15] However, hope is not easily defined or measurable. Generally speaking, "hope" may be defined as the "expectation of, or belief in, the fulfillment of something," but in a medical sense, particularly in the oncological world, hope means a great deal more. Hope is a value, provided it does not amount to an unrealistic optimism (which might stem from patients receiving misleading information or lacking awareness).[16]

Some studies describe the difference between realistic and unrealistic hopes. Realistic hopes are regarded as favorable elements for the patient,[17] while unrealistic hopes may be unfavorable, interfering with the correct compliance with treatments and concrete planning for the future. Even so, various studies have described hope as a fundamental positive factor while facing an oncological disease.[18] In general, then, realistic hope is to be considered a protective factor, while despair or a long-term despair may undermine the well-being and health of the patient.[19]

To tackle the issue of hope in a more rigorous way, some years ago we conducted a study aimed at investigating what and how hope was expressed within a cohort of cancer patients (of all ages) interviewed on a typical day at the Istituto Nazionale dei Tumori in Milan. The study was based on a self-administered questionnaire (developed by a team of physicians, psychologists, statisticians, and chaplains operating in various settings of the hospital). Since Italy is mainly a Christian country, it is important to underline that the theoretical model used to shape our questionnaire was Christian, but hope was interpreted as depending not only on religious aspects but also on psychological, spiritual, and relational dimensions. In all, 320 patients took part in the study (92.8 percent having a religious belief). Among the various collected findings, we may report:

- Women, patients with limited formal education, and believers were more hopeful.
- Patients placed trust variously in God, their partners and children, scientific research, and doctors.
- On univariate and multivariate analysis, patients' hope was related to their sharing of personal experiences with others (including family and friends), their positive perception of the people around them, and their relationship with doctors and nurses.

As a major conclusion, our study supports the notion that the quality of the relationship with caregivers affects the sense of hope of patients with cancer. This concept can be relevant for health care organization and resource allocation, as it underlines how hospitals need to be organized so as to enable relationships to happen, by suitably adjusting the workload or the numerical ratio of doctors to patients. In a further article reporting six specific clinical cases of adolescents, we described throughout the patients' dialogues how a chaplain can help young people to give voice to their emotions and thoughts about their sense of life and illness. Again, these experiences underlined how the constant presence of the chaplain in the multidisciplinary team, from the beginning of any treatment, can engender a good relationship with patients and help them keep hope and move forward.[20]

Announcing a poor prognosis or the beginning of a palliative care path to a severely ill, underage patient or the family of an underage patient is one of the most burdensome commitments a pediatric oncologist faces.[21] In this context, it essential to underline the importance of developing hope in the sense of illusion, which may help young patients face the extreme distress of the reality they are living, without removing their clinical situation.[22] Comparing the care experience of adolescents and adults with a poor prognosis, it is in fact interesting to note how, for adult patients, the possibility of organizing their work, their family, or their heritage may contribute to staying alive, to maintaining a sense of reality that forces them to remain active in ongoing life. The situation is different for an adolescent, who still needs to build his or her world and therefore needs to feel an adequate sense of idealization and illusion, though these realities are naturally affected by a serious disease.[23] Young adolescent patients who are severely ill or dying need to be able to talk to someone about their fear of dying, their nostalgia for all those things, and people they see moving further and further away from their grasp at an age that should be full of promise and dreams. The clinician must stay suspended alongside the patient and abstain from an interpretation that resolves this suspension.

Young people may often take an optimistic attitude to their clinical condition, still trusting in the future. We may sometimes wonder how adolescents in the advanced stages of cancer succeed in living a life that makes sense and what psychological mechanisms they rely on to do so. Little is known about the psychological processes implemented by terminal patients to react and adapt to reality. We believe that the rational sphere is not all-important. Within certain limits, at least, imagination can be a much more tolerable domain. In other words, a few illusions can have a positive effect, making reality more acceptable. Illusory defenses can avoid the anguish induced by thoughts of dying and prevent dissociative phenomena.

The doctor-patient relationship can, therefore, be characterized by building a suspension of the sense of reality in order to make everyday life tolerable. And while we know that there are harmful and dishonest deceptions, we also know that there are fundamental illusions that help build a livable sense of reality.

LUCIA'S DREAM

The delicate complexity of the power of illusion rises stunningly to the surface in the dream of a girl, Lucia, a seventeen-year-old patient with metastatic refractory soft-tissue sarcoma in terminal phase.[24] She tells the psychologist who works with adolescents on the ward:

"I had a strange dream. I haven't spoken about it to anyone, not even my mum or my best friend. I dreamt that I was at my eighteenth birthday party [a party that Lucia had been organizing for some time]. It was a fantastic party. I was dressed like a princess, in pale blue and white. Everyone was there, my parents, my brothers and sisters, my boyfriend, and all my friends. You doctors and nurses were there too, and all the other patients. Then at some point I saw Claudia [a

girl who had been with Lucia during numerous hospitalizations and many Youth Project activities, who had died not long beforehand]. Claudia looked lovely, but she was thin. I could see she was ill, and she couldn't talk. In my dream, I knew perfectly well that Claudia was dead, that she couldn't be there. But this didn't worry me. At some point, Claudia got into a hot-air balloon that was there, still attached to the ground, but that I knew would soon fly away. Her parents asked me if I could go with her because they didn't want her to leave alone. I really didn't want to leave the party, which was still in full swing. I was having a great time, and everyone was there for me. But, at the same time, I didn't want to leave Claudia alone. So I decided to go with her in the balloon. At some point, the balloon became detached from the ground and I began to rise up into the sky, higher and higher. I could see the party, and my friends and family, from above. I wasn't frightened, not at all, but I was very sorry to leave the people and the party behind. I already felt the loss. There was so much melancholy in my heart. I was sad, not frightened."

Lucia then said to the psychologist: "What do you think this dream means? To begin with, I was afraid it might mean I'm about to die. Then I realized that that's not it. There are still lots of therapies to try, and I've got lots of things to do: my eighteenth birthday party, a trip to the Caribbean, university. I think this dream meant to say that I can feel free to fly, to become light, freed of the weight of this difficult time, and even free to choose."

It is difficult to say whether Lucia's dream was true or not. That is beside the point because, by telling the story of her dream, Lucia was able to talk with the psychologist about her fear of dying, her trust in the future despite her clinical condition, her need to leave space for hope. This story shows the indispensable role of the imaginative sphere. Whether and how to tell a person who is terminally ill the truth about their condition remains a difficult issue. It is clear, however, that if such thoughts are experienced alone, they become intolerable. Still, it is not easy to talk about them, not even with loved ones—as Lucia said at the start of her story. These thoughts need to be shared with someone who is not afraid of them. Health care workers, including physicians, nurses, and chaplains, must be willing and able to fulfill this need; they must know how to listen. One of the many difficulties, of course, lies in knowing how to respond to an adolescent with terminal cancer, and there are no rules to define the best approach to use in daily clinical practice.

Still, by listening to adolescents, we are able to learn a great deal about health care. We learn about the need for health care institutes devoted exclusively to the needs of adolescents. We learn about the pivotal role played by attentive and compassionate caregivers, especially chaplains. We learn about the fundamental role of spirituality, even nascent spirituality. We learn about the impact of hope on health, even diminishing health. And we learn about the power of illusion. Mostly, we learn about life, about death, and about the inevitability of being suspended between them through Veronica's empathy, Chiara's dread, and Lucia's dream.

NOTES

1. Barr et al. 2016; Bleyer et al. 2008; Ferrari and Bleyer 2007; Ferrari 2014.
2. Ferrari et al. 2012.
3. Ibid.; Ferrari et al. 2016; Magni et al. 2016.
4. Veneroni et al. 2015; Ferrari et al. 2015; Ferrari, Gaggiotti, et al. 2017; Gaggiotti et al. 2019; Ferrari, Signoroni, et al. 2017b; Ferrari, Signoroni, et al. 2017a; Signoroni et al. 2019; Ferrari et al. 2019.
5. Veneroni et al. 2019.
6. Morgan et al. 2010; Marris, Morgan, and Stark 2011.
7. Halstead and Mickley 1997; Zinnbauer and Pargament 1998; Breitbart et al. 2004; Astrow et al. 2007.
8. Nicholas et al. 2017.
9. Marris, Morgan, and Stark 2011.
10. Proserpio et al. 2014.
11. Ibid.
12. Ibid.
13. Proserpio et al. 2016.
14. Pargament 1997; Fitzgerald Miller 2007.
15. Peteet and Balboni 2013; Montazeri 2009.
16. Proserpio et al. 2015.
17. Hilerman and Lackey 1990.
18. Enskär et al. 1997; Cantrell and Lupinacci 2004; Veneroni, Ferrari, Podda, et al. 2018.
19. Veneroni, Ferrari, Podda, et al. 2018.
20. Proserpio et al. 2020.
21. Stenmarker et al. 2010.
22. Veneroni, Ferrari, Prosperio, et al. 2018; Clerici et al. 2020.
23. Veneroni, Ferrari, Podda, et al. 2018.
24. Veneroni, Ferrari, Prosperio, et al. 2018.

WORKS CITED

Abrams, A. N., E. P. Hazen, and R. T. Penson. 2007. "Psychosocial Issues in Adolescents with Cancer." *Cancer Treatment Reviews* 33 (7): 622–30.

Astrow, A. B., A. Wexler, K. Texeira, M. K. He, D. P. Sulmasy. 2007. "Is Failure to Meet Spiritual Needs Associated with Cancer Patients' Perceptions of Quality of Care and Their Satisfaction with Care?" *Journal of Clinical Oncology* 25 (36): 5753–57.

Barr, R. D., A. Ferrari, L. Ries, J. Whelan, and W. A. Bleyer. 2016. "Cancer in Adolescents and Young Adults: A Narrative

Review of the Current Status and a View of the Future." *JAMA Pediatrics* 170 (5): 495–501.

Bleyer, A., R. Barr, B. Hayes-Lattin, D. Thomas, C. Ellis, B. Anderson, and Biology and Clinical Trials Subgroups of the U.S. National Cancer Institute Progress Review Group in Adolescent and Young Adult Oncology. 2008. "The Distinctive Biology of Cancer in Adolescents and Young Adults." *Nature Reviews Cancer* 8 (4): 288–98.

Breitbart, W., C. Gibson, S. R. Poppito, and A. Berg. 2004. "Psychotherapeutic

Interventions at the End of Life: A Focus on Meaning and Spirituality." *Canadian Journal of Psychiatry* 49 (6): 366–72.

Cantrell, M. A., and P. Lupinacci. 2004. "A Predictive Model of Hopefulness for Adolescents." *Journal of Adolescent Health* 35 (6): 478–85.

Clerici, C. A., E. Pagani Bagliacca, L. Veneroni, M. Podda, M. Silva, P. Gasparini, R. Luksch, M. Terenziani, M. Casanova, F. Spreafico, C. Meazza, V. Biassoni, E. Schiavello, S. Chiaravalli, T. Proserpio, M. Massimino, and A. Ferrari. 2020. "Adolescents with Terminal Cancer: Making Good Use of Illusions." *Journal of Adolescent and Young Adult Oncology* 9 (6): 683–86.

Enskär, K., M. Carlsson, M. Golsäter, and E. Hamrin. 1997. "Symptom Distress and Life Situation in Adolescents with Cancer." *Cancer Nursing* 20 (1): 23–33.

Ferrari, A. 2014. "SIAMO: Italian Pediatric Oncologists and Adult Medical Oncologists Join Forces for Adolescents with Cancer." *Pediatric Hematology and Oncology* 31 (6): 574–75.

Ferrari, A., and A. Bleyer. 2007. "Participation of Adolescents with Cancer in Clinical Trials." *Cancer Treatment Reviews* 33 (7): 603–8.

Ferrari, A., C. A. Clerici, M. Casanova, R. Luksch, M. Terenziani, F. Spreafico, D. Polastri, C. Meazza, L. Veneroni, S. Catania, E. Schiavello, V. Biassoni, M. Podda, and M. Massimino. 2012. "The Youth Project at the Istituto Nazionale Tumori in Milan." *Tumori* 98 (4): 399–407.

Ferrari, A., P. Gaggiotti, M. Silva, L. Veneroni, C. Magni, S. Signoroni, M. Casanova, R. Luksch, M. Terenziani, F. Spreafico, C. Meazzaa, C. A. Clerici, and M. Massimino. 2017. "Searching for Happiness." *Journal of Clinical Oncology* 35 (19): 2209–12.

Ferrari, A., S. Signoroni, M. Silva, P. Gaggiotti, L. Veneroni, C. A. Clerici, and M. Massimino. 2017a. "Viral! The Propagation of a Christmas Carol Produced by Adolescent Cancer Patients at the Istituto Nazionale Tumori in Milan, Italy." *Pediatric Blood and Cancer* 64 (9): e26516.

Ferrari, A., S. Signoroni, M. Silva, P. Gaggiotti, L. Veneroni, C. Magni, M. Casanova, S. Chiaravalli, M. Capelletti, P. Lapidari, C. A. Clerici, and M. Massimino. 2017b. "'Christmas Balls': A Christmas Carol by the Adolescent Cancer Patients of the Milan Youth Project." *Tumori* 103 (2): e9–e14.

Ferrari, A., M. Silva, L. Veneroni, C. Magni, C. A. Clerici, C. Meazza, M. Terenziani, F. Spreafico, S. Chiaravalli, M. Casanova, R. Luksch, S. Catania, E. Schiavello, V. Biassoni, M. Podda, L. Bergamaschi, N. Puma, A. Indini, T. Proserpio, and M. Massimino. 2016. "Measuring the Efficacy of a Project for Adolescents and Young Adults with Cancer: A Study from the Milan Youth Project." *Pediatric Blood and Cancer* 63 (12): 2197–204.

Ferrari, A., L. Veneroni, C. A. Clerici, M. Casanova, S. Chiaravalli, C. Magni, R. Luksch, M. Terenziani, F. Spreafico, D. Polastri, C. Meazz, S. Catania, E. Schiavello, V. Biassoni, M. Podda, L. Bergamaschi, N. Puma, C. Moscheo, G. Gotti, and M. Massimino. 2015. "Clouds of Oxygen: Adolescents with Cancer Tell Their Story in Music." *Journal of Clinical Oncology* 33 (2): 218–21.

Ferrari, A., L. Veneroni, S. Signoroni, M. Silva, P. Gaggiotti, M. Casanova, S. Chiaravalli, C. A. Clerici, T. Prosperio, and M. Massimino. 2019. "Loop: There's No Going Back: A Graphic Novel by Adolescent Cancer Patients on the Youth Project in Milan." *Journal of Medical Humanities* 4 (4): 505–11.

Fitzgerald Miller, J. 2007. "Hope: A Construct Central to Nursing." *Nursing Forum* 42 (1): 12–19.

Gaggiotti, P., L. Veneroni, S. Signoroni, M. Silva, M. Chisari, M. Casanova, S. Chiaravalli, G. Sironi, C. A. Clerici, T. Proserpio, M. Massimino, and A. Ferrari. 2019. "'What Shall I Do When I Grow Up?' Adolescents with Cancer on the Youth Project in Milan Play with Their Imagination and Photography." *Tumori* 105 (3): 193–98.

Halstead, M. T., and J. R. Mickley. 1997. "Attempting to Fathom the Unfathomable: Descriptive Views of Spirituality." *Seminars in Oncology Nursing* 13 (4): 225–30.

Hileman, J. W., and N. R. Lackey. 1990. "Self-Identified Needs of Patients with Cancer at Home and Their Home Caregivers: A Descriptive Study." *Oncology Nursing Forum* 17 (6): 907–13.

Magni, C., L. Veneroni, M. Silva, M. Casanova, S. Chiaravalli, M. Massimino, C. A. Clerici, and A. Ferrari. 2016. "Model of Care for Adolescents and Young Adults with Cancer: The Youth Project in Milan." *Frontiers in Pediatrics* 4 (August): 88.

Marris, S., S. Morgan, D. Stark. 2011. "'Listening to Patients': What Is the Value of Age-Appropriate Care to Teenagers and Young Adults with Cancer?" *European Journal of Cancer Care* 20 (2): 145–51.

Montazeri, A. 2009. "Quality of Life Data as Prognostic Indicators of Survival in Cancer Patients: An Overview of the Literature from 1982 to 2008." *Health and Quality of Life Outcomes* 7:102.

Morgan, S., S. Davies, S. Palmer, and M. Plaster. 2010. "Sex, Drugs, and Rock 'n' Roll: Caring for Adolescents and Young Adults with Cancer." *Journal of Clinical Oncology* 28 (32): 4825–30.

Nicholas, D. B., M. Barrera, L. Granek, N. M. D'Agostino, J. Shaheed, L. Beaune, E. Bouffet, and B. Antle. 2017. "Parental Spirituality in Life-Threatening Pediatric Cancer." *Journal of Psychosocial Oncology* 35 (3): 323–34.

Pargament, K. I. 1997. *The Psychology of Religion and Coping: Theory, Research, Practice.* New York: Guilford Press.

Peteet, J. R., and M. Balboni. 2013. "Spirituality and Religion in Oncology." *CA: A Cancer Journal for Clinicians* 63 (4): 280–89.

Proserpio, T., A. Ferrari, S. Lo Vullo, M. Massimino, C. A. Clerici, L. Veneroni, C. Bresciani, P. G. Casali, M. Ferrri, P. Bossi, G. Galmozzi, A. Pierantozzi, L. Licitra, S. Marceglia, and L. Mariani. 2015. "Hope in Cancer Patients: The Relational Domain as a Crucial Factor." *Tumori* 101 (4): 447–54.

Proserpio, T., A. Ferrari, L. Veneroni, C. Arice, M. Massimino, and C. A. Clerici. 2018. "Cooperation Between In-Hospital Psychological Support and Pastoral Care Providers: Obstacles and Opportunities for a Modern Approach." *Tumori* 104 (4): 243–51.

Proserpio, T., A. Ferrari, L. Veneroni, B. Giacon, M. Massimino, and C. A. Clerici. 2014. "Spiritual Aspects of Care for Adolescents with Cancer." *Tumori* 100 (4): 130e–35e.

Proserpio, T., E. Pagani Bagliacca, G. Sironi, C. A. Clerici, L. Veneroni, M. Massimino, and A. Ferrari. 2020. "Spirituality and Sustaining Hope in Adolescents with Cancer: The Patients' View." *Journal of Adolescent and Young Adult Oncology* 9 (1): 36–40.

Proserpio, T., L. Veneroni, M. Silva, A. Lassaletta, R. Lorenzo, C. Magni, M. Bertolotti, E. Barisone, M. Mascarin, M. Jankovic, P. D'Angelo, C. A. Clerici, C. Garrido-Colino, I. Gutierrez-Carrasco, A. Echebarria, A. Biondi, M. Massimino, F. Casale, A. Tamburini, and A. Ferrari. 2016. "Spiritual Support for Adolescent Cancer Patients: A Survey of Pediatric Oncology Centers in Italy and Spain." *Tumori* 102 (4): 376–80.

Signoroni, S., L. Veneroni, E. Pagani Bagliacca, P. Gaggiotti, M. Silva, M. Casanova, S. Chiaravalli, C. A. Clerici, M. Massimino, and A. Ferrari. 2019. "'Summer Is You': Adolescents and Young Adults with Cancer Sing About Their Desire for Summer." *Pediatric Blood and Cancer* 66 (5): e27630.

Stenmarker, M., U. Hallberg, K. Palmérus, and I. Márky. 2010. "Being a Messenger of Life-Threatening Conditions: Experiences of Pediatric Oncologists." *Pediatric Blood and Cancer* 55 (3): 478–84.

Veneroni, L., C. A. Clerici, T. Proserpio, C. Magni, G. Sironi, S. Chiaravalli, L. Roncari, M. Casanova, L. Gandola, M. Massimino, and A. Ferrari. 2015. "Creating Beauty: The Experience of a Fashion Collection Prepared by

Adolescent Patients at a Pediatric Oncology Unit." *Tumori* 101 (6): 626–30.

Veneroni, L., A. Ferrari, M. Podda, T. Proserpio, E. Pagani Bagliacca, M. Massimino, and C. A. Clerici. 2018. "About the Good Use of Illusions in Oncology: End-of-Life Experiences and Communications in Adolescent Patients." *Recenti progressi in medicina* 109 (3): 166–73.

Veneroni, L., A. Ferrari, T. Proserpio, E. Pagani Bagliacca, M. Podda, M. Massimino, and C. A. Clerici. 2018. "Dreams and Illusions in Adolescents with Terminal Cancer." *Tumori* 104 (6): 413–14.

Veneroni, L., P. Gaggiotti, D. Ciceri, E. Rosati, M. Massimino, and A. Ferrari. 2019. "From the Seventh Floor to Seventh Heaven." *Tumori* 105 (6): 529–30.

Zebrack, B., and S. Isaacson. 2012. "Psychosocial Care of Adolescent and Young Adult Patients with Cancer and Survivors." *Journal of Clinical Oncology* 30 (11): 1221–26.

Zinnbauer, B. J., and K. I. Pargament. 1998. "Spiritual Conversion: A Study of Religious Change Among College Students." *Journal for the Scientific Study of Religion* 37 (1): 161–80.

Appendix

The Marialuisa Lectureship for Life
A Brief Introduction

Mauro Ferrari

The genesis of this volume can be traced to the Marialuisa Lectureship for Life. These lectures are the epicenter of activity that eventually led the Vatican to host the Palliative Care and Spirituality for Life conference at Houston Methodist Hospital, in collaboration with the University of Texas MD Anderson Cancer Center, in September of 2018.

There is a poignant history to these lectures. Marialuisa Fusello Ferrari died at age thirty-two on September 18, 1994, in Berkeley, California. She died in intractable pain, derived from gynecological cancer with visceral metastases. She was survived by me—her husband—and three children: Giacomo, then six years old, and twin sisters Kim and Chiara, then four years old. I later remarried Paola del Zotto; we had twin girls, Ilaria and Federica, and Paola adopted Giacomo, Kim, and Chiara.

Our family determined, as soon as financial resources were available, to honor Marialuisa. The opportunity emerged in 1999, when I became one of the first two researchers to receive the Wallace H. Coulter Award for Innovation and Entrepreneurship, administered by the Georgia Institute of Technology. The Coulter Award carried with it a stipend of $100,000, so I consulted with my dear friend at Ohio State University, an anesthesiologist specializing in symptom control and palliative medicine, Costantino Benedetti, who has contributed to this volume. Nino and I discussed the marvelous ways in which the money could be put to use. After a few conversations resulting in the purchase of a Suburban, acquired to brave frigid Ohio winters with a growing family and affectionately named the "Coulter-mobile," I agreed to endow part of the stipend for the Marialuisa Ferrari Lectureship for Life. Further resources were later contributed by George and Tina Skestos at the Ohio State University, as well as Houston Methodist Hospital, the University of Texas MD Anderson Cancer Center, McGovern Medical School at UT Health, the University of St. Thomas in Houston, our family, and numerous other private donors.

The purpose of the Marialuisa Lectureship for Life is, in essence, to fight cancer-related pain and the broader range of life-threatening symptoms of cancer and to contribute to the discovery of relevant remedies for pain and suffering wherever they occur. These commitments are evident in the lectureship's dedication, which I wrote at the time of Marialuisa's death; these commitments are reproduced in the plaques that honor Marialuisa lecturers:

> Marialuisa—all lives in your smile,
> All unraveling mysteries
> The abyss of cessation
> And the continuity of Light.
> The needlessness of pain—'tis our promise—
> And us with you,
> Turning screaming tears into peaceful murmurs of times,
> And meanings,
> And the caress of infinities,
> Divine.

Over the years, the Marialuisa Lectureship was awarded to an extraordinary set of accomplished individuals who have dedicated their lives to goals that are harmonious with the objectives of the lecture. The first three lecturers, Neil MacDonald, Kathleen Foley, and Declan Walsh, two of whose essays are included in this volume, are founders of contemporary palliative medicine, especially with respect to oncology. The next year, Andrew von Eschenbach, former director of the National Cancer Institute and commissioner of the Food and Drug Administration, spoke of the necessity for early intervention against pain in cancer care as a more effective antidote than many current pharmaceutical treatments against metastatic disease. Edmund Pellegrino, a leader in the field of biomedical ethics, reflected upon the ethical requirement of providing palliation for pain.

During the years 2005 to 2008, lecturers focused upon various dimensions of the ethical mandate to serve patients holistically. Nobel laureate Richard Smalley was unable to deliver his lecture in person, as he lay dying of his own cancer, though he delivered his remarks, in an affecting and effective gesture, virtually; these were accompanied by a panel convened to discuss the transformational breakthroughs in cancer care that were on the horizon through nanotechnology—a field he had pioneered—and other inventive approaches. Next came Frances M. Visco, founder and president of the National Breast Cancer Coalition, who spoke about the extraordinary power of patient advocacy in the fight for health care advances. The following year, TV anchor turned patient-rights activist Mino Damato vividly chronicled the inhumane treatment of abandoned HIV-infected children in Ceaușescu's Romanian orphanages, which Damato likened to concentration camps. Breast cancer surgeon Umberto Veronesi, the original developer of quadrantectomies in breast cancer, reflected upon the decades-long pathway he took, against considerable resistance, to bring his novel surgical procedure to millions of cancer-stricken women.

During the next four years, beginning in 2009, the lectureship revisited themes of palliative medicine from the perspective of global leaders from a variety of disciplines. Ben Rich championed broad educational improvements in the delivery of supportive care. Eduardo Bruera described the model palliative care center he established at MD Anderson. Linda Emanuel delivered an ethical framework for the role of chaplains in palliative care. Allan Basbaum surveyed the state of the art in the science of pain and its care.

For more than a decade, Costantino Benedetti had chaired the awards committee for the Marialuisa Lectureship for Life. In 2013, the committee orchestrated a benign takeover in order to invite Nino, a champion and practitioner of palliative and pain medicine, to deliver the lecture. Benedetti was forthright, arguing that the denial of adequate pain medication is tantamount to a deprivation of basic human rights and dignity. In 2014, Philip A. Pizzo detailed the position of the expert panel on pain medicine of the National Academy of Medicine (then the National Institute of Medicine of the National Academy of Sciences), which he had chaired. The following year, philanthropist and community leader in London Sir Thomas Hughes-Hallett discussed the opportunities he had been given to influence end-of-life care standards in the United Kingdom and globally.

In 2016, the Marialuisa Lectureship for Life took place in coordination with one held at the Houston Methodist Hospital and another at the original site, the Ohio State University. Two individuals received posthumous awards: Giovanni (John) Bonica, a founder of palliative medicine in the United States, and Arthur James, a leading oncologist at the Ohio State University, after whom its cancer center is named. In a parallel event, the Houston-based lecture was delivered by Joseph Fins, leading neurologist and bioethicist—and yet another contributor to this volume—who focused upon the human rights of minimally conscious patients.

In successive years, Tony Yaksh and Charles von Gunten delivered lectures on the campus of the Ohio State University. In Houston, American football professional Devon Still spoke about support for children with cancer; he reflected upon his own experience of caring for his daughter, Leah, who, diagnosed with a neurological form of cancer at age five, survived the ordeals of diagnosis and treatment.

The final Marialuisa Lectureship was presented in honor of His Holiness, Pope Francis, at the opening of the Palliative Care and Spirituality for Life conference, which provided the impetus for this book. Pope Francis sent a letter of thanks and blessing to Marialuisa, my family, and those embroiled in the effort to palliate pain; this letter now graces the wall of the home of Marialuisa's mother, Caterina, in Udine, Italy. Monsignor Vincenzo Paglia, president of the Pontifical Academy for Life, who had read the letter aloud, delivered a lecture in which he underscored the moral responsibility of an equitable distribution of relief against suffering worldwide. He traced the association of the Pontifical Academy with palliative medicine, particularly in the poorest regions in the world. This mandate, that call, provides an appropriate conclusion to the first two decades of the Marialuisa Lectureship for Life and an apt précis of this volume, which recounts groundbreaking efforts of early palliativists, ethical challenges faced in palliative care, spiritual dimensions of those who suffer, and the highest ideals not of palliative care alone but of attentive and intelligent care, period.

THE MARIALUISA LECTURESHIP FOR LIFE: SPEAKERS AND TITLES, 2000–2018

2018
Nineteenth Annual Marialuisa Lectureship for Life
Houston Methodist Award Recipient—His Eminence Archbishop Vincenzo Paglia and the Pontifical Academy for Life, In Honor of the Holy Father, Pope Francis
The Ohio State University Award Recipient— Charles von Gunten, MD, PhD, FAAHPM, FAACE | OhioHealth, Riverside Methodist Hospital
Taking Palliative Care Mainstream: A Glimpse of the Future
2017
Houston Methodist Award Recipient—Devon Still | Still Strong Foundation
A Father's Experience Tackling Childhood Cancer
The Ohio State University Award Recipient— Tony Yaksh, PhD | University of California San Diego
Frontiers in Pain Research
2016—Joseph J. Fins, MD, MACP | Cornell University Weill Cornell Medicine
Preserving the Right to Die and Affirming the Right to Care
The Ohio State University Award Recipient— Arthur G. James, MD (posthumous) | The Ohio State University; and John J. Bonica, MD (posthumous) | University of Washington
2015—Sir Thomas Hughes-Hallett | Imperial College and Chelsea-Westminster Hospital, London, UK
How Philanthropy and Social Entrepreneurship Can Transform the Care of the Dying
2014—Philip A. Pizzo, MD | Stanford University
Chronic Pain: Overcoming a Public Health Challenge
2013—Costantino Benedetti, MD | The Ohio State University and International Association for the Study of Pain
The Two Faces of Pain: A Beneficial, Warning Vital Function; A Malefic, Consuming Neurologic Disease
2012—Allan Basbaum, PhD | University of California San Francisco
Can We Treat the "Disease" of Neuropathic Pain

2011—Linda Emanuel, MD, PhD | Northwestern University
The Last Frontier in Palliative Care Research: Bringing Rigor to Research in Palliative Care Chaplaincy
2010—Eduardo Bruera, MD, FAAHPM | The University of Texas MD Anderson Cancer Center
Palliative Cancer Care for Patients and Healthcare Professionals
2009—Ben A. Rich, JD, PhD | University of California Davis
Palliative Care Education and the Culpability of Cultivated Ignorance
2008—Umberto Veronesi | Istituto Europeo Oncologia
New Paradigms in the Management of Breast Cancer
2007—Mino Damato | Bambini in Emergenza
The Unknown Odyssey of Abandoned Children with HIV
2006—Frances M. Visco | National Breast Cancer Coalition
The Power of Patient Advocacy
2005—Richard Smalley, MD | Rice University
Hope on the Cancer Front
2004—Edmund D. Pellegrino, MD, MACP | Georgetown University
Palliative Care: Some Ethical Considerations
2003—Andrew C. von Eschenbach, MD | Samaritan Health Initiatives Inc.
Palliative Care as a Cancer Intervention: Progress with a Purpose
2002—T. Declan Walsh, MD | Levine Cancer Institute, Carolinas HealthCare System
Palliative Medicine in Modern Cancer Care
2001—Kathleen M. Foley, MD | Cornell University Weill Cornell Medicine
Improving Palliative Care for Cancer: A National Cancer Policy Board Report
2000—Neil MacDonald, MD | University of Alberta and McGill University
Integrating Palliative Care into Oncology Practice

W. Andrew Achenbaum, PhD, is Professor Emeritus at the Texas Medical Center. He previously was Professor of History and Deputy Director of the Institute of Gerontology at the University of Michigan and Founding Dean of the College of Liberal Arts and Social Sciences at the University of Houston. A recipient of the Gerontological Society of America's Kent Award, Achenbaum formerly chaired the National Council of Aging.

Stacy L. Auld, MDiv, serves as the Director of Spiritual Care and Values Integration at Houston Methodist Hospital in Houston, Texas. She is an ordained elder in the Texas Annual Conference of The United Methodist Church and a board-certified chaplain and member of the Association of Professional Chaplains.

Elena Pagani Bagliacca, DPsych, is a psychologist and psychotherapist who has worked for years with adult and pediatric cancer patients. She has been one of the psychologists dedicated to adolescents of the Youth Project in Milan.

Costantino Benedetti, MD, FAAPM, is a graduate of the University of Rome. The recipient of an NIH fellowship in pain medicine at the University of Washington and mentored by John Bonica and Richard Chapman, he joined the Department of Anesthesiology. In 1990, he joined the James Cancer Hospital at the Ohio State University to develop a cancer pain and symptom control program. Benedetti considers the bequest of Bonica's personal medical library his most valued recognition.

Courtenay R. Bruce, MA, JD, is director of system patient experience for the Houston Methodist Hospital System. She is an attorney, mediator, researcher, and ethicist. Her research and publications focus on clinician-to-patient communication and surrogate decision-making, along with the use and effectiveness of patient-centered digital technologies.

Eduardo Bruera, MD, FAAHPM, is the Chair of the Department of Palliative, Rehabilitation and Integrative Medicine at the University of Texas MD Anderson Cancer Center. His clinical interest is the care of the physical and psychosocial distress of patients with cancer and their families. He has more than one thousand peer-reviewed publications and has edited thirty-one books. He has received multiple federal research grants in the United States and Canada, as well as a number of national and international awards.

Joseph Calandrino, MA, DO, FAAFP, CAQ after over thirty years of practicing general medicine, geriatrics, and hospice and palliative medicine, recently retired from clinical medicine, though he remains a faculty member of the Renaissance School of Medicine in SUNY Stony Brook, New York. He continues to read and write in phenomenology, and he is currently composing curricula on the philosophy and ethics of the body for undergraduate and graduate students.

James Cleary, MD, professor and Walther Senior Chair of Supportive Oncology at Indiana University School of Medicine, serves as Director of Supportive Oncology and Medical Director, IU Simon Comprehensive Cancer Center. Trained in medical oncology in Australia, Cleary works to improve cancer care and pain relief globally. The American Academy of Hospice and Palliative Care recognized him as a global visionary in palliative care; he received the 2021 Floriani Award from the European Association of Palliative Care.

Constance Dahlin, MSN, ANP-BC, ACHPN', FPCN, FAAN, is a board-certified palliative care specialist. She developed hospice in the urban and community setting and palliative care in the community, academic, and clinic settings. She is a clinician, educator, administrator, author, and consultant within palliative care. She has served on various national committees and work groups; authored peer-reviewed articles, chapters, and curricula; and presented nationally and internationally.

Andrea Ferrari, MD, has worked since 1994 at the Pediatric Oncology Unit of the Istituto Nazionale dei Tumori of Milan. He has had numerous leadership positions in international cooperative groups dedicated to soft-tissue sarcomas (European Pediatric Soft Tissue Sarcoma Study Group, EpSSG) and pediatric rare tumors (European Cooperative Study Group for Pediatric

Rare Tumors, ExPERT). He works with the Youth Project in Milan and chairs various scientific organizations devoted to oncology and adolescents.

Mauro Ferrari, PhD, is Professor of Pharmaceutics at the University of Washington. He has held faculty appointments in engineering and medicine at the University of California, Berkeley, the Ohio State University, the University of Texas Medical School, MD Anderson Cancer Center, Houston Methodist Hospital, and Weill Cornell Medical College. He received his MS and PhD degrees in mechanical engineering at Berkeley and a degree in mathematics from the University of Padova, Italy.

Robert Fine, MD, FACP, FAAHPM, is the Director of Clinical Ethics and Supportive Palliative Care at Baylor Scott and White Health. He was intimately involved in the creation of the Texas Advance Directives Act and has served as an ethics consultant for both national and regional health care organizations. He serves on the editorial board of the *Journal of Pain and Symptom Management*, teaches, and publishes widely in ethics and palliative care with a particular focus on medical futility.

Joseph J. Fins, MD, MACP, FRCP, is the E. William Davis, Jr. M.D. Professor of Medical Ethics, Professor of Medicine, and Chief, Division of Medical Ethics at Weill Cornell Medicine. At Yale Law School he is the Solomon Center Distinguished Scholar in Medicine, Bioethics and the Law and Visiting Professor of Law.

Bettie Jo Tennon Hightower, DMin, served as Senior Staff Chaplain for Houston Methodist Hospital. She began her thirty-eight-year affiliation with hospitals as a registered nurse in the operating room. Driven by the findings of her doctoral study on helping individuals find meaning in their life experiences, she successfully championed the need for a full-time chaplain on the palliative care team. She is a pastor, theologian, and life coach.

Kathryn B. Kirkland, MD, holds the Dorothy and John J. Byrne, Jr. Distinguished Chair in Palliative Medicine at the Geisel School of Medicine and chief of Palliative Medicine at Dartmouth-Hitchcock Health. In addition to her clinical practice, she facilitates activities in humanities and narrative medicine, including cross-disciplinary activities with colleagues at Dartmouth

College, and integrates narrative medicine teaching into medical student, resident, faculty, and healthcare team education.

John R. (Jack) Levison, PhD, holds the W. J. A. Power Chair of Old Testament Interpretation and Biblical Hebrew at Perkins School of Theology, Southern Methodist University. Jack has done research at St. Andrews University, Eberhard-Karls-Universität Tübingen, Ludwig-Maximilians-Universität München, and Oxford Brookes University. He has received fellowships from the National Humanities Center, the Alexander von Humboldt Foundation, the International Catacomb Society, the Louisville Institute, the Lilly Endowment, and the Rotary Foundation.

Robin W. Lovin, PhD, is Cary M. Maguire University Professor of Ethics Emeritus at Southern Methodist University and a Visiting Scholar in Theology at Loyola University Chicago. He joined the Southern Methodist University faculty in 1994, and served as Dean of the Perkins School of Theology from 1994 to 2002. His books include *Christian Realism and the New Realities* and *An Introduction to Christian Ethics*, and he is coeditor of the *Oxford Handbook of Reinhold Niebuhr*.

Neil MacDonald, MD, CM, FRCP(C), FRCP (Edinburgh Honorary), LLD (University of Calgary Honorary), is Emeritus Professor at the University of Alberta and McGill University. A protégé of Balfour Mount, MacDonald was coeditor of the first two editions of the *Oxford Textbook of Palliative Medicine*, coeditor of *Palliative Medicine: A Case-Based Manual*, Secretary-Treasurer of the American Society of Clinical Oncology, a member of the 1997 Institute of Medicine Report on Care at the End of Life, and director of the Cross Cancer Institute, University of Alberta.

Charles R. Millikan, DMin, is the Vice President for Spiritual Care and Values Integration for Houston Methodist Hospital and holds the Dr. Ronny W. and Ruth Ann Barner Centennial Chair of Spiritual Care. He is also a Clinical Professor in the Center for Medical Ethics and Health Policy at the Baylor College of Medicine and an Adjunct Professor with the Perkins School of Theology at Southern Methodist University. He is also a retired Elder in the Texas Annual Conference of The United Methodist Church.

Dominique J. Monlezun, MD, PhD, PhD, MPH, is a practicing physician–data scientist and philosopher who seeks to heal humanity through ethical and equitable artificial intelligence. He is Principal Investigator and Senior Data Scientist for over one hundred research studies, Professor of Bioethics for two United Nations–affiliated universities, Adjunct Professor of Cardiovascular Medicine for the University of Texas system, and author of the first textbook on integral ethical AI.

Tullio Proserpio, STD, graduated from the Psychology Institute of the Pontificia Università Gregoriana, Rome, and gained qualifications in pastoral health at the Pontificia Università Lateranense, Rome, including training in counseling and hospital-based work. He has been chaplain at the Istituto di Ricerca e Cura a Carattere Scientifico (IRCCS), in collaboration with the Istituto Nazionale dei Tumori of Milan, since 2003. He works daily with the pediatric department and participates in Youth Project meetings.

Giovanna Sironi, MD, is a pediatrician working at the Pediatric Oncology Unit of the Istituto Nazionale dei Tumori of Milan. She graduated in medicine and completed her pediatric residency at the Università degli Studi di Milano, focusing on pediatric oncology.

Daniel P. Sulmasy, MD, PhD, MACP, is the André Hellegers Professor of Biomedical Ethics in the Departments of Medicine and Philosophy and Director of the Kennedy Institute of Ethics at Georgetown University. A practicing internist and a philosopher, he has written extensively about medical ethics and the spirituality of medical care. His seven books include *The Healer's Calling, The Rebirth of the Clinic, Methods in Medical Ethics,* and *Euthanasia and Assisted Suicide: Before, During, and After the Holocaust.*

Declan Walsh, MD, MSc, FACP, FRCP, holds the Hemby Chair of Supportive Oncology at the Levine Cancer Institute. Walsh graduated from University College Dublin and did a medical oncology/pharmacology fellowship at Memorial Sloan Kettering Cancer Center. In 1987, he started the first palliative medicine program in the United States. His honors include a visionary award from the American Academy of Hospice and Palliative Medicine and a lifetime achievement award from the Multinational Association for Supportive Care in Cancer.